Crisis Standards of Care

A Toolkit for Indicators and Triggers

Committee on Crisis Standards of Care: A Toolkit for Indicators and Triggers

Board on Health Sciences Policy

Dan Hanfling, John L. Hick, and Clare Stroud, *Editors*

INSTITUTE OF MEDICINE
OF THE NATIONAL ACADEMIES

THE NATIONAL ACADEMIES PRESS
Washington, D.C.
www.nap.edu

THE NATIONAL ACADEMIES PRESS   500 Fifth Street, NW   Washington, DC 20001

NOTICE: The project that is the subject of this report was approved by the Governing Board of the National Research Council, whose members are drawn from the councils of the National Academy of Sciences, the National Academy of Engineering, and the Institute of Medicine. The members of the committee responsible for the report were chosen for their special competences and with regard for appropriate balance.

This study was supported by Contract No. HHSP23337003T between the National Academy of Sciences and the Department of Health and Human Services and Contract No. DTNH22-10-H-00287 between the National Academy of Sciences and the Department of Transportation's National Highway Traffic Safety Administration. Any opinions, findings, conclusions, or recommendations expressed in this publication are those of the author(s) and do not necessarily reflect the views of the organizations or agencies that provided support for the project.

International Standard Book Number-13:   978-0-309-28552-0
International Standard Book Number-10:   0-309-28552-6

Additional copies of this report are available for sale from the National Academies Press, 500 Fifth Street, NW, Keck 360, Washington, DC 20001; (800) 624-6242 or (202) 334-3313; http://www.nap.edu.

For more information about the Institute of Medicine, visit the IOM home page at: **www.iom.edu.**

The serpent has been a symbol of long life, healing, and knowledge among almost all cultures and religions since the beginning of recorded history. The serpent adopted as a logotype by the Institute of Medicine is a relief carving from ancient Greece, now held by the Staatliche Museen in Berlin.

Suggested citation: IOM (Institute of Medicine). 2013. *Crisis standards of care: A toolkit for indicators and triggers.* Washington, DC: The National Academies Press.

"Knowing is not enough; we must apply.
Willing is not enough; we must do."
—Goethe

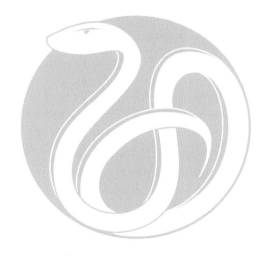

INSTITUTE OF MEDICINE
OF THE NATIONAL ACADEMIES

Advising the Nation. Improving Health.

THE NATIONAL ACADEMIES
Advisers to the Nation on Science, Engineering, and Medicine

The **National Academy of Sciences** is a private, nonprofit, self-perpetuating society of distinguished scholars engaged in scientific and engineering research, dedicated to the furtherance of science and technology and to their use for the general welfare. Upon the authority of the charter granted to it by the Congress in 1863, the Academy has a mandate that requires it to advise the federal government on scientific and technical matters. Dr. Ralph J. Cicerone is president of the National Academy of Sciences.

The **National Academy of Engineering** was established in 1964, under the charter of the National Academy of Sciences, as a parallel organization of outstanding engineers. It is autonomous in its administration and in the selection of its members, sharing with the National Academy of Sciences the responsibility for advising the federal government. The National Academy of Engineering also sponsors engineering programs aimed at meeting national needs, encourages education and research, and recognizes the superior achievements of engineers. Dr. C. D. Mote, Jr., is president of the National Academy of Engineering.

The **Institute of Medicine** was established in 1970 by the National Academy of Sciences to secure the services of eminent members of appropriate professions in the examination of policy matters pertaining to the health of the public. The Institute acts under the responsibility given to the National Academy of Sciences by its congressional charter to be an adviser to the federal government and, upon its own initiative, to identify issues of medical care, research, and education. Dr. Harvey V. Fineberg is president of the Institute of Medicine.

The **National Research Council** was organized by the National Academy of Sciences in 1916 to associate the broad community of science and technology with the Academy's purposes of furthering knowledge and advising the federal government. Functioning in accordance with general policies determined by the Academy, the Council has become the principal operating agency of both the National Academy of Sciences and the National Academy of Engineering in providing services to the government, the public, and the scientific and engineering communities. The Council is administered jointly by both Academies and the Institute of Medicine. Dr. Ralph J. Cicerone and Dr. C. D. Mote, Jr., are chair and vice chair, respectively, of the National Research Council.

www.national-academies.org

COMMITTEE ON CRISIS STANDARDS OF CARE: A TOOLKIT FOR INDICATORS AND TRIGGERS

DAN HANFLING (*Co-Chair*), Inova Health System, Falls Church, VA
JOHN L. HICK (*Co-Chair*), Hennepin County Medical Center, Minneapolis, MN
SARITA CHUNG, Harvard School of Medicine and Boston Children's Hospital, MA
CAROL CUNNINGHAM, Ohio Department of Public Safety, Columbus
BRIAN FLYNN, Uniformed Services University of the Health Sciences, Bethesda, MD
W. NIM KIDD, Texas Department of Public Safety, Austin
ANN R. KNEBEL, National Institute of Nursing Research, National Institutes of Health, Bethesda, MD
LINDA SCOTT, Michigan Department of Community Health, Lansing
ANTHONY H. SPEIER, State of Louisiana's Department of Health and Hospitals, Baton Rouge
JOLENE R. WHITNEY, Bureau of Emergency Medical Services and Preparedness, Utah Department of Health, Salt Lake City

IOM Staff

CLARE STROUD, Study Director
BRUCE M. ALTEVOGT, Senior Program Officer
SHEENA M. POSEY NORRIS, Research Associate
DOUGLAS KANOVSKY, Senior Program Assistant
LORA TAYLOR, Financial Associate
DONNA RANDALL, Administrative Assistant
ANDREW M. POPE, Director, Board on Health Sciences Policy

Reviewers

This report has been reviewed in draft form by individuals chosen for their diverse perspectives and technical expertise, in accordance with procedures approved by the National Research Council's Report Review Committee. The purpose of this independent review is to provide candid and critical comments that will assist the institution in making its published report as sound as possible and to ensure that the report meets institutional standards for objectivity, evidence, and responsiveness to the study charge. The review comments and draft manuscript remain confidential to protect the integrity of the deliberative process. We wish to thank the following individuals for their review of this report:

Hany Abdelaal, VNSNY CHOICE Health Plans
Knox Andress, Louisiana Poison Center
Tracy Buchman, HSS, Inc.
Barbara B. Citarella, RBC Limited
Peggy Connorton, American Health Care Association
Nancy W. Dickey, Texas A&M Health Science Center
Chris Kelenske, Michigan State Police
Arthur L. Kellermann, RAND Corporation
Danita Koehler, Governor's Alaska Council on Emergency Medical Services
Deborah Levy, Centers for Disease Control and Prevention
Onora Lien, Northwest Healthcare Response Network
Suzet McKinney, Chicago Department of Public Health
Ann Norwood, Center for Biosecurity of UPMC
Sarah Park, Hawaii Department of Health
Nels Sanddal, American College of Surgeons
Leslee Stein-Spencer, National Association of State EMS Officials

Although the reviewers listed above have provided many constructive comments and suggestions, they were not asked to endorse the conclusions or recommendations nor did they see the final draft of the report before its release. The review of this report was overseen by **Mark R. Cullen,** Stanford University. Appointed by the Institute of Medicine, he was responsible for making certain that an independent examination of this report was carried out in accordance with institutional procedures and that all review comments were carefully considered. Responsibility for the final content of this report rests entirely with the authoring committee and the institution.

Contents

User Guide

This report focuses on *indicators* (measurements or predictors of change in demand for health care services or availability of resources) and *triggers* (decision points about adaptations to health care service delivery) that guide operational decision making about providing care during public health and medical emergencies and disasters. It includes a discussion toolkit designed to facilitate discussions about indicators and triggers within and across health care organizations, health care coalitions, emergency response agencies, and jurisdictions. This report builds on previous Institute of Medicine reports on crisis standards of care, including *Guidance for Establishing Crisis Standards of Care for Use in Disaster Situations* (2009) and *Crisis Standards of Care: A Systems Framework for Catastrophic Disaster Response* (2012).

The report is divided into two parts; it is possible to start with either part, depending on the reader's goals:

To review background information about crisis standards of care and explore concepts related to indicators and triggers, start by reading Chapters 1 and 2.

To jump directly into the discussion toolkit, start with Chapter 3, which provides the introduction to the toolkit and material relevant to the entire emergency response system. Then proceed to the chapter corresponding to the component of the emergency response system of greatest interest: emergency management (Chapter 4), public health (Chapter 5), behavioral health (Chapter 6), emergency medical services (Chapter 7), hospital and acute care (Chapter 8), and out-of-hospital care (Chapter 9). Because integrated planning across the emergency response system is critical for a coordinated response, it is important to read the toolkit introduction (Chapter 3) as well as the discipline-specific chapters.

Acronyms

ALS	advanced life support
ASPR	Assistant Secretary for Preparedness and Response
BARDA	Biomedical Advanced Research and Development Authority
BH	behavioral health
BLS	basic life support
CDC	Centers for Disease Control and Prevention
COP	Common Operating Picture
CSC	crisis standards of care
DHS	Department of Homeland Security
DMAT	Disaster Medical Assistance Team
DMORT	Disaster Mortuary Operational Response Team
DMRU	Disaster Medical Response Unit
DoD	Department of Defense
EAP	employee assistance program
ED	emergency department
EMAC	Emergency Management Assistance Compact
EMS	emergency medical services
EOC	emergency operations center
ESAR-VHP	Emergency System for Advance Registration of Volunteer Health Professionals
ESF	Emergency Support Function
FEMA	Federal Emergency Management Agency
FQHC	federally qualified health center
GFT	Google Flu Trends

HAN	Health Alert Network
HCC	health care coalition
HCF	health care facility
HCO	health care organization
HHS	Department of Health and Human Services
HICS	Hospital Incident Command System
HIPAA	Health Insurance Portability and Accountability Act
HPP	Hospital Preparedness Program
HRSA	Health Resources and Services Administration
HVA	Hazard Vulnerability Analysis
IC	incident command
ICU	intensive care unit
ILI	influenza-like illness
IMSURT	International Medical Surgical Response Team
IOM	Institute of Medicine
JIC	Joint Information Center
LTC	long-term care
MAA	mutual aid agreement
MAC	Medical Advisory Committee
MAC	multiagency coordination
MCI	mass casualty incident
MOU	Memorandum of Understanding
MRC	Medical Reserve Corps
MSCC	Medical Surge Capacity and Capability
MSSS	Michigan Syndromic Surveillance System
MTF	Military Treatment Facility
NASEMSO	National Association of State EMS Officials
NCIPC	National Center for Injury Prevention and Control
NDMS	National Disaster Medical System
NEDOCS	Naitonal Emergency Department Overcrowding Score
NHTSA	National Highway Traffic Safety Administration
NIMS	National Incident Management System
NN	no notice
NVRT	National Veterinary Response Team
NWS	National Weather Service

PACU	postanesthesia care unit
PFA	psychological first aid
PH	public health
PHEP	Public Health Emergency Preparedness
POD	point of dispensing
PPE	personal protective equipment
RDMAC	Regional Disaster Medical Advisory Committee
RMCC	Regional Medical Coordination Center
SARS	severe acute respiratory syndrome
SDMAC	State Disaster Medical Advisory Committee
SEOC	state emergency operations center
SME	subject matter expert
SNS	Strategic National Stockpile
SO	slow onset
SOFA	Sequential Organ Failure Assessment
VA	Department of Veterans Affairs
VAMC	U.S. Department of Veterans Affairs Medical Center

Summary

Disasters such as Hurricane Katrina, Hurricane Sandy, the earthquake in Haiti, and the tornado in Joplin, Missouri, have served as vivid reminders of the challenge of providing health care when demand for health care services sharply rises and places overwhelming demand on resources and medical staff, all in the midst of infrastructure damage or destruction. Severe pandemic influenza or catastrophic terrorist incidents—such as the detonation of a nuclear device or the release of a bioterrorism agent—have the potential to place even greater demands on the health system.

Planning to provide care in these types of overwhelming situations can help health care organizations and providers, supported by the entire emergency response system, take proactive steps that enable them to provide patients with the level of care they would usually receive, or care that is functionally equivalent, for as long as possible. In catastrophic disasters, however, these proactive steps may become insufficient: health care resources may become so scarce that reallocation decisions are needed, staff may have to practice outside of their normal scope of practice, and the focus of patient care may need to switch to promoting benefits to the population over benefits to individuals. In this austere situation, planning is necessary to avoid greater illness, injury, and death by enabling more effective use of the limited resources through fair, just, and equitable processes for making decisions about who should receive treatments when there are not enough resources to provide patients with the level of care they would usually receive. Recent incidents such as the Boston bombing and the tornado in Moore, Oklahoma, have demonstrated the value of notification, planning, and exercising in avoiding what could have been far greater illness, injury, and death. The response to these incidents also emphasized the importance of a network of resources to absorb the demands of major incidents.

Decision making about the level of care that can be provided during a disaster is important and complex. Health care organizations and providers should not prematurely move to providing care that presents a risk of a compromised outcome to patients, but at the same time they should take proactive steps to use resources carefully if demand is expected to surge and/or resource shortages are anticipated. The amount of information available in health care today is enormous, and expanding, and determining how to use it to inform operational decision making is both challenging and critical. Information may be incomplete and contradictory; it is collected and stored by many different entities; it can be challenging to detect or characterize an emerging event amid usual variability in large and complex sets of data; forecasting demand is difficult; and decisions must be made in a novel, urgent, dynamic, and often chaotic set of circumstances.

Over the past decade, federal, state, tribal, and local governments, the Institute of Medicine (IOM), and other entities have embarked on developing crisis standards of care (CSC) plans and guidance. As this body of work continues to evolve, the need for guidance on how to develop indicators and triggers that aid decision making about the provision of care in disasters has been identified as a gap. Indicators are measurements or predictors of change in demand for health care service delivery or availability of resources. An example indicator could be *emergency department wait time*. Triggers are decision points that are based on changes in the availability of resources that require adaptations to health care services delivery along the care continuum.[1] An example trigger could be *emergency department wait time exceeds X hours*, which would trigger a variety of response tactics such as increased staffing.

Advance planning about indicators and triggers involves considering what information about demand and resources is available across the health care spectrum (from prehospital to end-of-life care), how this information is shared and integrated, how this information drives actions, and what actions might be taken to provide the best health care possible given the situation. Because of the stress, complexity, and uncertainty inherent in a crisis situation, it is particularly important that these conversations occur in advance. Planning for indicators and triggers has to occur at the level of the specific organization, agency, or community, because it depends on the usual resources and demand. For example, a tornado that touches down in a small, rural community may automatically warrant activation of the health care organization disaster plan, whereas additional information about the size and location of the tornado may be required before making this decision in a larger community with a higher ability to absorb a surge in demand.

At the request of the Assistant Secretary for Preparedness and Response at the Department of Health and Human Services, the National Highway Traffic Safety Administration in the Department of Transportation, and the Veterans Health Administration, in the fall of 2012 the IOM convened the Committee on Crisis Standards of Care: A Toolkit for Indicators and Triggers. The task was to prepare a conversation toolkit to guide stakeholders through the process of developing indicators and triggers that may govern the transition across the continuum of care, from *conventional* standards of care to *contingency* surge response and standards of care to *crisis* surge response and standards of care, and back to *conventional* standards of care.

REPORT DESIGN AND ORGANIZATION

Chapter 1 provides background on crisis standards of care. Chapter 2 discusses key concepts, limitations, and systems-level considerations related to developing indicators and triggers. Chapters 3-9 constitute a discussion toolkit designed to help stakeholders have discussions about indicators and triggers. Chapter 3 provides the overarching framework for the toolkit and should be read by everyone. Chapters 4 through 9 are customized for each major component of the emergency response system: emergency management (Chapter 4), public health (Chapter 5), behavioral health (Chapter 6), emergency medical services (EMS) (Chapter 7), hospital and acute care (Chapter 8), and out-of-hospital care (Chapter 9).[2] Because

---

[1] "The surge capacity following a mass casualty incident falls into three basic categories, depending on the magnitude of the incident: conventional, contingency, and crisis. These categories also represent a corresponding continuum of patient care delivered during a disaster. As the imbalance increases between resource availability and demand, health care—emblematic of the health care system as a whole—maximizes conventional capacity; then moves into contingency; and, once that capacity is maximized, moves finally into crisis capacity. A crisis situation may lead to an overwhelming demand for services and result in shortages of equipment, supplies, pharmaceuticals, personnel, and other critical resources, necessitating operational adjustments" (IOM, 2012, p. 1-6)

[2] The out-of-hospital care delivery system includes diverse ambulatory care environments (public, private, tribal, veterans health, military), home health and hospice, assisted living and skilled nursing, specialty care and resources, and others.

what occurs in one of the emergency response disciplines is likely to affect, or be affected by, what occurs in other components of the emergency response system, readers should read the chapter(s) specific to their discipline and also review the other chapters.

BACKGROUND ON CRISIS STANDARDS OF CARE

This report builds on two previous IOM reports on crisis standards of care: *Guidance for Establishing Crisis Standards of Care for Use in Disaster Situations* (2009), which presented key concepts related to CSC, and *Crisis Standards of Care: A Systems Framework for Catastrophic Disaster Response* (2012), which further developed an operational framework for planning for and implementing CSC. This section briefly summarizes concepts from these two reports, focusing on those that are essential to understanding the approach taken in this report.

Both reports emphasize the importance of developing indicators and triggers in CSC plans. The 2009 report described five key elements that should underlie all CSC plans:

1. A strong ethical grounding that enables a process deemed equitable and just based on its transparency, consistency, proportionality, and accountability;
2. Integrated and ongoing community and provider engagement, education, and communication;
3. The necessary legal authority and legal environment in which CSC can be ethically and optimally implemented;
4. *Clear indicators*, *triggers*, and lines of responsibility; and
5. Evidence-based clinical processes and operations.

These reports also emphasized the need to continually monitor demand and resources, and to strive to move back toward conventional care as quickly as feasible.

A Systems Approach to Catastrophic Disaster Response

Successfully responding to a catastrophic disaster will require integrated planning, coordination, cooperation, consultation, and follow-through among many response disciplines and agencies, including state and local governments, EMS, health care coalitions, health care organizations, and health care providers in the community. The 2012 report developed a systems framework for catastrophic disaster response, which includes, but is not limited to, the development and implementation of CSC plans. In this framework, ethical considerations and the legal authority and environment form the foundation that undergirds crisis standards of care planning and implementation. A number of key elements underlie the development of CSC plans, including provider engagement, community engagement, *development of indicators and triggers*, implementation of clinical processes, and operations. Education and information sharing are the cornerstones of the framework; together with the process of performance improvement, they support the key elements of CSC planning and enable midcourse corrections during the implementation of the framework. The systems framework has five pillars of medical surge: hospital care, public health, out-of-hospital care, emergency medical services, and emergency management and public safety. To ensure a unified disaster response, these different components of the disaster response system need to be well integrated. The final components of the systems framework are the federal, state, tribal and territorial, and local governments, which have an overarching responsibility for the development, institution, integration, and proper execution of CSC plans, policies, protocols, and procedures.

Integrated planning within and across a tiered system of relationships among individual health care organizations, health care coalitions, and local, state, and federal governments is critical for a coordinated response and to avoid prematurely moving to a different level of response along the continuum of care that may adversely impact patient care. The Medical Surge Capacity and Capability framework outlines such a tiered system, and the 2012 IOM report integrates CSC planning and implementation into this framework (Barbera and Macintyre, 2007, 2009; IOM, 2012). As described below, the toolkit is designed to support discussions at all tiers in this system and among all components of the emergency response system.

Continuum of Care: Conventional, Contingency, and Crisis

Rather than just focusing on the most extreme circumstances, the committee that authored the 2009 and 2012 reports, as well as the current committee, envision surge capacity as occurring along a continuum based on resource availability and demand for health care services. One end of this continuum is defined by conventional care, which describes services that are provided in health care organizations on a routine or daily basis. In the middle of the continuum, contingency care provides care that is functionally equivalent to usual patient care (e.g., one medication substituted for another that is not usually used in that circumstance but provides the same or a similar effect). At the far end of the continuum is crisis care, when the best possible care is provided to the population of patients as a whole because of the very limited resources available. Significant changes are made in the methods and locations of care delivery, and decision making shifts from patient-centered to population-centered outcomes.

It is important to recognize that transitions along the continuum of care do not always occur abruptly. For example, a slow-onset incident such as an influenza pandemic may result in a relatively gradual transition through the continuum, while an improvised nuclear device detonation near a downtown medical center may require an immediate transition to crisis care. Along this continuum, indicators demonstrate the potential for movement toward a different level of care: from conventional to contingency, from contingency to crisis, or from crisis back toward conventional. The triggers are decision points, based on changes in the availability of resources, which require adaptations to health care services delivery along the care continuum. In this report, triggers that lead to the implementation of crisis standards of care have been specifically designated as *crisis care triggers* because this is the point at which resource allocation strategies focus on the community rather than the individual, carrying the greatest potential adverse impact to patient outcomes; the implementation of crisis standards of care at this point aims to minimize adverse patient outcomes to the extent possible given the circumstances and available resources.

INDICATORS AND TRIGGERS

Indicators and triggers represent the information and actions taken at specific thresholds that guide incident *recognition*, *response*, and *recovery*. When specific indicators cross a threshold that is recognized by the community to require action, this represents a trigger point, with actions determined by community plans. These include activation of a general disaster plan, which often occurs at the threshold between conventional and contingency care, or activation of CSC plans, which would occur at the threshold between contingency and crisis care.

Developing Useful Indicators and Triggers

It is attractive to look at many of the metrics available in health care today and consider their use as indicators. However, multiple factors may make data monitoring less useful than it originally appears, and it can be complex to detect actionable information or an evolving event amid usual variability in large sets of data. Specific numeric thresholds for indicators and triggers are concrete and attractive because they are easily recognized. For certain situations they are relatively easy to develop (e.g., a single case of anthrax), but for many situations the community/agency actions are not as clear-cut or may require significant data analysis to determine where a reasonable threshold may be established (e.g., multiple cases of diarrheal illness in a community).

The report outlines key concepts related to indicators, data, triggers, and tactics that will help inform decisions about how best to develop and use them. Depending on the nature of the indicator and data, different types of triggers and tactics may be required.

Actionable and predictive indicators: Actionable indicators *can* be impacted through actions taken within an organization or a component of the emergency response system (e.g., a hospital detecting high patient census). *Predictive* indicators *cannot* be impacted through actions taken within a health care organization or other component of the emergency response system (e.g., a hospital receiving notification that a pandemic virus has been detected may lead to the implementation of response tactics, but the indicator is considered *predictive* because the hospital's actions cannot impact or reverse the virus having been detected).

Indicators are comprised of data, broadly understood to include measurements, predictions, or events (for example, a 911 call or witnessing a tornado). Data may be *certain* or *uncertain: Certain* data require minimal validation or analysis (e.g., temperature, emergency department wait times), allowing rapid decision making and lending themselves more readily to the assignment of discrete thresholds at which a trigger is implemented. *Uncertain* data require interpretation to determine the appropriate response; triggers based on uncertain data may involve expert analysis before action. An important note is that decision making in crises often requires acting on uncertain information. The fact that information is uncertain means that additional assessment and analysis may be required, but this should not impede the ability to plan and act.

Scripted and non-scripted triggers: Scripted triggers are decision points that require minimal analysis and lead to scripted tactics. *Non-scripted* triggers are decision points that require analysis and lead to implementation of non-scripted tactics.

Scripted and non-scripted tactics: Scripted tactics are a predefined action or set of actions that are easily and quickly implemented by frontline personnel. *Non-scripted* tactics vary according to the situation; they are based on analysis of multiple inputs, recommendations, and, in certain circumstances, previous experience, and are tailored to the requirements of the situation.

Actionable indicators comprised of certain data can often appropriately lead to scripted triggers and tactics; examples of this would be a hospital trauma team activation or a first alarm response to a report of fire in a building. With some exceptions, predictive indicators, usually comprised of uncertain data, most appropriately lead to non-scripted triggers and tactics. An example would be the decision-making process leading to the declaration of an influenza pandemic. Regardless of the certainty of the data, each pathway requires a "filter" process in which information is analyzed, assessed, and verified. With certain data, this filter process may be minimal. These concepts are illustrated in Figure S-1.

When developing plans for indicators and triggers, stakeholders should keep in mind the following types of limitations and issues associated with indicators: the accuracy of the data being used as an indicator; naming conventions and "rules of reporting," particularly when indicators are being shared among multiple entities (e.g., to determine how many intensive care unit beds are available in a city, it will be important to know whether hospitals are counting and reporting only staffed beds or currently unstaffed beds as well); the dynamic environment in which data are reported; and the challenge of detecting evolving changes amid usual data variability. When developing plans for indicators and triggers, the time required for an entity to report data may detract from response efforts. Automating the information exchange, where possible,

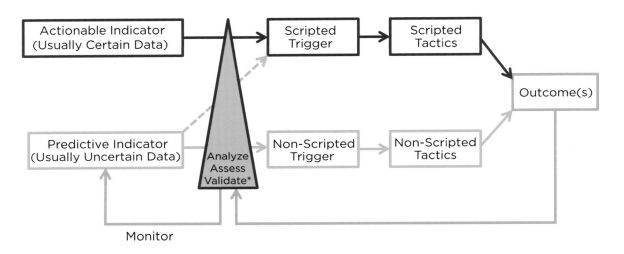

FIGURE S-1
Relationships among indicators, triggers, and tactics.
*Interpret indicators, other available data, impact, and resources—this may occur over minutes (e.g., developing an initial response to a fire) or days (e.g., developing a response to the detection of a novel virus).
NOTE: In this figure, an indicator is comprised of either certain data, sufficient to activate a trigger, or uncertain data, which require additional analysis prior to action. It is important to note several characteristics that may be helpful in shaping planning:

- All actions require at least minimal validation of data or processing of data—the triangle at the center of the figure shows the relative amount of processing expertise and time required (i.e., the thicker base of the triangle represents more processing required).
- Indicators that are actionable typically involve certain data that can lead to scripted triggers that staff can initiate without further analysis (e.g., if a mass casualty incident involves >20 victims, the mass casualty incident [MCI] plan is activated).
- Indicators that are predictive (e.g., epidemiology data) typically involve uncertain data that require interpretation prior to "trigger" action.
- The smaller the community or the fewer resources available, the more certain and scripted the triggers can become.
- The larger the community (or state/national level) and the more resources available, the less certain the data become as they do not reflect significant variability in resource availability at the local level—thus, the more expert interpretation is often required prior to action (e.g., state level data may reveal available beds, but select facilities and/or jurisdictions may be far beyond conventional capacity).
- The larger or more direct the impact, the more certain the data (e.g., when the tornado hits your hospital, there is no question you should trigger your disaster plan and implement contingency or crisis care tactics as required).
- Scripted triggers are quickly implemented by frontline personnel with minimal analysis—the disadvantage is that the scripted tactics may commit too few or too many resources to the incident (e.g., first alarm response to report of a fire in a building).
- Non-scripted triggers are based on expert analysis rather than a specific threshold and allow implementation of tactics that are tailored to the situation (non-scripted tactics). Trigger decisions may be based on expertise, experience, indicator(s) interpretation, etc., and may be made quickly or take significant time based on the information available.
- Ongoing monitoring and additional analysis of indicators will help assess the current situation and the impact of the tactics.

is valuable. To avoid making unnecessary requests for information, an important consideration is how the information will drive specific operational decisions and actions.

Return to Conventional Care

As conditions improve, it is important to watch for indicators that the system can move back toward conventional care status. These indicators may be incident specific and not included in an agency's usual data or list of indicators. Examples of these indicators may include decreasing call or emergency department volumes, restored systems (utilities, etc.), and decreasing use of hotlines and dispensing sites. These indicators may fluctuate over the course of a disaster response, so return to conventional may be temporary. Return to conventional care status is not the same as recovery, although it may be an indicator of transition into the recovery phase. Recovery implies a more permanent return to normal operating status and the restoration of the impacted systems and communities.

Systems-Level Considerations

Integrated planning among all major components of the emergency response system is critical for an effective and coordinated response. Integrated planning for indicators and triggers also needs to occur among these components of the system, both horizontally and vertically. In addition to thinking about limitations and issues inherently associated with the indicators themselves, it is important to think about how the information will be shared and synthesized and used by different components of the emergency response system.

DISCUSSION TOOLKIT

The objective of the toolkit is to facilitate discussions about indicators and triggers within and across health care organizations, health care coalitions, emergency response agencies, and jurisdictions. Specifically, the toolkit focuses on indicators and triggers that guide transitions along the continuum of care, from *conventional* standards of care to *contingency* surge response and standards of care to *crisis* surge response and standards of care, and back to *conventional* standards of care. Agencies and stakeholders should understand what information is available to support operational decision making in this kind of situation, and what triggers may automatically activate particular responses or may require expert analysis prior to a decision. This toolkit is intended to help agencies and stakeholders have these discussions. The outcomes of these discussions can be used to drive policy, planning, and exercises.

Toolkit Design

The discussion toolkit is structured around two scenarios (one slow-onset and one no-notice), a series of key questions for discussion, and a set of example tables. The example indicators and triggers encompass both clinical and administrative domains.

Chapter 3 provides the introduction to the toolkit and material relevant to the entire emergency response system, including the scenarios, a set of key overarching questions, and example indicators, triggers, and tactics related to worker functional capacity, an important crosscutting issue for all components of the emergency response system. The second part of the toolkit is provided in Chapters 4 through 9, which are each aimed at a key component of the emergency response system: emergency management, public health, behavioral health, EMS, hospital and acute care, and out-of-hospital care. These chapters provide additional questions intended to help participants drill down on the key issues for their own discipline. These chapters also contain tables that provide example indicators, triggers, and tactics across the continuum of care, followed by a blank table for participants to complete. The scenarios, questions, and example table are intended to help facilitate discussion that would result in completing the blank table. The examples provided are not exhaustive and are just intended as examples. The tables need to be discussed and developed at the organization, agency, and jurisdiction levels because of variability in daily resource availability, demand, infrastructure, information sources, and actions that may be taken.

This toolkit has been designed to be scalable for use at multiple levels. Discussions need to occur at the facility, organization, and agency levels to reflect the level of detail about organizational capabilities needed for operational decision making. Discussions also need to occur at higher tiers of the emergency response system to ensure regional consistency and integration; it is important to understand the situation in other organizations and components of the emergency response system to avoid prematurely moving to a more austere level of care when resources might be available elsewhere.

For communities that have already begun CSC planning, this toolkit can be used to develop or expand the indicator and trigger components of their plan. For communities that are beginning the CSC planning process, the use of this toolkit—and the exploration of community-, regional-, and state-derived indicators, triggers, and the process by which actions are then taken—would be an excellent place to start this important work. The toolkit discussions will provide much of the needed detailed understanding about what it means to transition away from conventional response and toward the delivery of health care that occurs in contingency conditions, or in worst cases, under crisis conditions. For additional guidance on the development of CSC plans, including planning milestones and templates, see the IOM's 2012 report.

These discussions will provide a foundation for future policy work, planning, and exercises related to CSC planning and disaster planning in general. The indicators and triggers developed for CSC planning purposes are subject to change over time as planned resources become more or less available or circumstances change. It will be important to regularly review and update CSC plans, including indicators and triggers.

REFERENCES

Barbera, J. A., and A. G. Macintyre. 2007. *Medical surge capacity and capability: A management system for integrating medical and health resources during large-scale emergencies,* 2nd ed. Washington, DC: U.S. Department of Health and Human Services. http://www.phe.gov/preparedness/planning/mscc/handbook/documents/mscc080626.pdf (accessed April 3, 2013).

Barbera, J. A., and A. G. Macintyre. 2009. *Medical surge capacity and capability: The healthcare coalition in emergency response and recovery.* Washington, DC: U.S. Department of Health and Human Services. http://www.phe.gov/preparedness/planning/mscc/documents/mscctier2jan2010.pdf (accessed May 14, 2013).

IOM (Institute of Medicine). 2009. *Guidance for establishing crisis standards of care for use in disaster situations: A letter report.* Washington, DC: The National Academies Press.

IOM. 2012. *Crisis standards of care: A systems framework for catastrophic disaster response.* Washington, DC: The National Academies Press.

1: Introduction

Over the past decade, federal, state, tribal, and local governments, the Institute of Medicine (IOM), and other entities have embarked on developing crisis standards of care (CSC) plans and guidance (e.g., AHRQ, 2005; Devereaux et al., 2008; IOM, 2009, 2012; Ohio Hospital Association and Ohio Department of Health, 2011; Phillips and Knebel, 2007; State of Michigan, 2013; Timbie et al., 2012). CSC planning is intended to help the emergency response system—including emergency management, public health, behavioral health, emergency medical services (EMS), health care organizations and providers—provide patients with the best care possible given the circumstances. In catastrophic disasters involving an overwhelming demand for medical care, CSC planning is also intended to enable more effective use of the limited resources through fair, just, and equitable processes for making decisions about who should receive treatments when there are not enough resources to provide patients with the level of care they would usually receive.

As this body of work continues to evolve, the need for guidance on how to incorporate indicators and triggers that aid decision making about the provision of care in disasters has been identified as a gap. Indicators are measurements or predictors of change in demand for health care service delivery or availability of resources. Triggers are decision points that are based on changes in the availability of resources that require adaptations to health care services delivery along the care continuum.[1] Advance planning about indicators and triggers involves considering what information about demand and resources is available across the health care spectrum, how this information is shared and integrated, how this information drives actions, and what actions might be taken to provide the best health care possible given the situation. Because of the stress, complexity, uncertainty, and time sensitivity inherent in a crisis situation, it is important that these discussions occur in advance. The development and use of indicators and triggers helps enable good decision making.

This report provides an overview of key considerations relevant to the development of indicators and triggers and a toolkit designed to facilitate discussions among stakeholders in developing indicators and triggers for their own organizations, agencies, regional health care coalitions, and states. The toolkit provides

---

[1] "The surge capacity following a mass casualty incident falls into three basic categories, depending on the magnitude of the incident: conventional, contingency, and crisis. These categories also represent a corresponding continuum of patient care delivered during a disaster. As the imbalance increases between resource availability and demand, health care—emblematic of the health care system as a whole—maximizes conventional capacity; then moves into contingency; and, once that capacity is maximized, moves finally into crisis capacity. A crisis situation may lead to an overwhelming demand for services and result in shortages of equipment, supplies, pharmaceuticals, personnel, and other critical resources, necessitating operational adjustments" (IOM, 2012, p. 1-6)

key questions and example indicators and triggers for the major components of the emergency response system: emergency management, public health, behavioral health, EMS, hospital and acute care, and out-of-hospital. The toolkit is designed to be scalable for use at multiple levels, from the facility, organization, and agency levels up through the whole community's emergency response system. Discussions need to occur at all levels so they include the level of detail about organizational capabilities that is needed for operational decision making, within the context of integrative planning for a coordinated response. These discussions will help the stakeholders develop the capabilities described in both the Hospital Preparedness Program (HPP) and the Public Health Emergency Preparedness (PHEP) cooperative agreements (ASPR, 2012a; CDC, 2011).

STUDY GOALS AND METHODS

At the request of the Assistant Secretary for Preparedness and Response (ASPR) at the Department of Health and Human Services (HHS), the National Highway Traffic Safety Administration (NHTSA) in the Department of Transportation, and the Veterans Health Administration, in the fall of 2012 the IOM convened the Committee on Crisis Standards of Care: A Toolkit for Indicators and Triggers. The task was to prepare a conversation toolkit to guide stakeholders through the process of developing indicators and triggers that may govern their health system's transition across the continuum of care, from *conventional* standards of care to *contingency* surge response and standards of care to *crisis* surge response and standards of care, and back to *conventional* standards of care. Box 1-1 presents the statement of task.

This committee was made up of experts in the fields and sectors responsible for implementing CSC, including public health, emergency medicine, nursing, pediatrics, EMS, emergency management, and disaster behavioral health. Appendix C contains biosketches of the committee members. The work of the current committee builds on the work of a previous IOM committee, the Committee on Guidance for Establishing Standards of Care for Use in Disaster Situations (IOM, 2009, 2012). The work of that committee is described below.

To gather stakeholder input, the current committee held an open meeting in January 2013. Panelists from different stakeholder perspectives were invited, including public health, emergency management, EMS, health care coalitions, home health, long-term care and nursing homes, behavioral health, specialty burn care, and information management. The committee also sought input on the task from representatives of the federal government, including ASPR and NHTSA. The committee met in closed session in conjunction with the open meeting and once again in March 2013 to review the evidence and draft the report.

In addition, the committee reviewed relevant literature. The MEDLINE/PubMed and Scopus databases were searched using the following terms (in a variety of combinations): *indicator, metric, measure, trigger, predictor, warning, precipitating factors, health system indicator, health system trigger,* and *health system measure,* combined with the terms *disaster, surge capacity, surge capability, medical surge, crisis standards of care,* and *allocation of scarce resources.*[2] Abstracts were reviewed and selected for relevance to the topic at hand. Finally, the committee examined previous efforts to determine indicators and triggers in publicly available state and local crisis standards of care plans.

---

[2] The committee would like to thank Alicia Livinski of the National Institutes of Health Library for her help in conducting these searches.

ORGANIZATION OF THE REPORT AND HOW TO USE THE TOOLKIT

This chapter provides a brief introduction to the concepts in crisis standards of care that are particularly relevant to indicators and triggers, as well as a discussion of the importance of developing indicators and triggers. This chapter summarizes certain key concepts from earlier IOM work on crisis standards of care. These reports contain extensive information and resources about developing CSC plans, including templates for planning and implementing CSC (IOM, 2009, 2012). These reports also cover in more detail key areas that are outside of the scope of full discussion in this report, including legal, ethical, and palliative care issues.

Chapter 2 discusses how to develop useful indicators and triggers, limitations and issues associated with indicators, and systems-level issues related to indicators and triggers. Chapters 3 through 9 form the toolkit. Chapter 3 provides the overarching framework for the toolkit and should be read first by everyone. Chapters 4 through 9 are customized for each component of the emergency response system: emergency management (Chapter 4), public health (Chapter 5), behavioral health (Chapter 6), EMS (Chapter 7), hospital and acute care (Chapter 8), and out-of-hospital care (Chapter 9). Because integrated planning across the emergency response system is critical for a coordinated response, it is important to read the toolkit introduction (Chapter 3) as well as the discipline-specific chapters.

This toolkit aims to provide the basis for discussions about indicators and triggers, and includes example indicators and triggers that are intended to help stakeholders start discussions specific to their own situations rather than serve as definitive lists. Indicators and triggers need to be discussed and developed at the agency, jurisdiction, and regional levels because of variability in daily resource availability and demand, infrastructure and available information, and actions that may be taken in response to an indicator or a trigger. The toolkit should be used to facilitate planning discussions in advance of a disaster so these discussions can occur without the stress, complexity, uncertainty, and time pressure of a disaster situation.

The discussion toolkit is structured around two scenarios, a series of key questions for discussion, and a set of example tables. The example indicators and triggers encompass both clinical and administrative indicators and triggers. The committee included two scenarios (one slow-onset [influenza pandemic] and one no-notice incident [earthquake]) to make the discussions more vivid and to stimulate discussion. The scenarios also serve to help participants achieve an understanding of what the different components of the emergency response system would be facing during a catastrophic disaster and what they would be focused on, providing a necessary common picture to support discussions across these components. Scenario-based planning is the first component of the "hybrid planning approach" that is strongly advocated by the Federal Emergency Management Agency (FEMA) in its comprehensive preparedness guide and also described as the approach that health and public health planners commonly use (ASPR, 2012a; FEMA, 2010). This approach was also used in the recent discussion guides on pandemic influenza planning that were prepared at the request of the Centers for Disease Control and Prevention (ORISE 2013a,b,c).

PREVIOUS IOM WORK ON CRISIS STANDARDS OF CARE

During the spring of 2009, the IOM's Forum on Medical and Public Health Preparedness for Catastrophic Events hosted a series of regional meetings on crisis standards of care. These regional meetings were intended to build on early work in this area, including efforts by the Government Accountability Office, the Agency for Healthcare Research and Quality, the New York State Task Force on Life and the Law, and the American College of Chest Physicians Task Force for Mass Critical Care (AHRQ, 2005; Devereaux et al., 2008; GAO, 2008; Powell et al., 2008). Discussions at the regional meetings identified the development of national guidance on standards of care during disaster situations as a crucial area for improving the nation's preparedness (IOM, 2010).

Later that year, in the midst of the 2009 H1N1 pandemic, the ASPR asked the IOM to convene a committee of experts to develop guidance that health officials could use to establish and implement standards of care during disasters. The resulting letter report defined crisis standards of care as

> A substantial change in usual health care operations and the level of care it is possible to deliver, which is made necessary by a pervasive (e.g., pandemic influenza) or catastrophic (e.g., earthquake, hurricane) disaster. This change in the level of care delivered is justified by specific circumstances and is formally declared by a state government in recognition that crisis operations will be in effect for a sustained period. The formal declaration that crisis standards of care are in operation enables specific legal/regulatory powers and protections for health care providers in the necessary tasks of allocating and using scarce medical resources and implementing alternate care facility operations. (IOM, 2009, p. 3)[3]

The report also described five key elements that should underlie all CSC plans:

1. A strong ethical grounding that enables a process deemed equitable and just based on its transparency, consistency, proportionality, and accountability;
2. Integrated and ongoing community and provider engagement, education, and communication;

---

[3] The 2009 and 2012 reports emphasize the importance of the state's role and of appropriate state declaration to recognize the need for crisis standards of care. However, it is also important that disaster planning, including planning for CSC, occur at all levels. Particularly in a no-notice disaster, the transition to crisis may need to be implemented immediately, although an appropriate declaration should be made as soon as possible and/or the authorities of the state director of public health should be used to implement actions (where applicable and appropriate).

3. The necessary legal authority and legal environment in which CSC can be ethically and optimally implemented;
4. Clear indicators, triggers, and lines of responsibility; and
5. Evidence-based clinical processes and operations.

In 2010, ASPR, the Department of Veterans Affairs (VA), and NHTSA asked the IOM expert committee to reconvene to provide concepts and guidance to help state and local officials apply the CSC framework the committee created earlier. In its 2012 report, *Crisis Standards of Care: A Systems Framework for Catastrophic Disaster Response*, the committee examined the effect of its 2009 report, and developed underlying principles, concepts, planning milestones, and templates to guide the efforts of professionals and organizations responsible for CSC planning and implementation (IOM, 2012).[4] Like all of the IOM CSC work, this report took an all-hazards approach. The 2009 and 2012 reports have been referred to in HHS's Hospital Preparedness Program and Public Health Emergency Preparedness cooperative agreements (ASPR, 2012a; CDC, 2011).

The following sections present key concepts from the 2009 and 2012 reports, with a specific focus on those that are relevant to indicators and triggers.

CONTINUUM OF CARE: CONVENTIONAL, CONTINGENCY, AND CRISIS

Rather than focusing exclusively on the most extreme circumstances, the committee that authored the 2009 and 2012 reports, as well as the current committee, envision surge capacity as occurring along a continuum based on resource availability and demand for health care services. One end of this continuum is defined by conventional care, which describes services that are provided in health care organizations on a daily basis. In the middle of the continuum, contingency care provides care that is functionally equivalent to usual patient care (e.g., one medication substituted for another that is not usually used in that circumstance but provides the same or a similar effect). At the far end of the continuum is crisis care, when the best possible care is provided to the population of patients as a whole because of the very limited resources available. Changes are made in the methods and locations of care delivery that present significant increased risk of adverse outcomes, and decision making shifts from patient-centered to population-centered outcomes. These levels of care are described in Box 1-2. Figure 1-1 illustrates how a surge response may shift across the continuum from conventional to crisis care based on the demand and supply mismatch that may occur over time, particularly as it affects the availability of patient care spaces; staff; and needed supplies, equipment, and pharmaceuticals.

A key observation is that transitions along the continuum of care do not always occur abruptly. For example, a slow-onset incident such as an influenza pandemic may result in a relatively gradual transition through the continuum, while an improvised nuclear device detonation near a downtown medical center may require an immediate transition to crisis care. Along this continuum, indicators demonstrate the potential for movement toward a different level of care: from conventional to contingency, from contingency to

---

[4] The 2012 report and associated materials are available at http://www.iom.edu/crisisstandards.

BOX 1-2
Conventional, Contingency, and Crisis Care

Conventional capacity: The spaces, staff, and supplies used are consistent with daily practices within the institution. These spaces and practices are used during a major mass casualty incident that triggers activation of the facility emergency operations plan.

Contingency capacity: The spaces, staff, and supplies used are not consistent with daily practices, but provide care that is *functionally equivalent* to usual patient care. These spaces or practices may be used temporarily during a major mass casualty incident or on a more sustained basis during a disaster (when the demands of the incident exceed community resources).

Crisis capacity: Adaptive spaces, staff, and supplies are not consistent with usual standards of care, but provide sufficiency of care in the context of a catastrophic disaster (i.e., provide the best possible care to patients given the circumstances and resources available). Crisis capacity activation constitutes a significant adjustment to standards of care.

SOURCE: Hick et al., 2009.

---

crisis, or from crisis back toward conventional.[5] The triggers are decision points, based on changes in the availability of resources, which require adaptations to health care services delivery along the care continuum.

A SYSTEMS APPROACH TO CATASTROPHIC DISASTER RESPONSE

Successfully responding to a catastrophic disaster will require integrated planning, coordination, cooperation, and consultation of many response disciplines and agencies, including state and local governments, EMS, health care organizations, and health care providers in the community. The 2012 report developed a systems framework for catastrophic disaster response, which includes, but is not limited to, the development and implementation of CSC plans.[6] This framework is illustrated in Figure 1-2; certain elements are discussed briefly below, but much greater detail is available in the 2012 report.[7]

In this framework, ethical considerations and the legal authority and environment form the foundation. As emphasized in both the 2009 and 2012 reports, it is critical that ethical decision making underlies all

---

[5] The 2009 and 2012 reports described indicators as being those data points occurring at the boundary of conventional to contingency care that demonstrated the potential for movement toward crisis standards of care. These reports focused on triggers as delineating the movement into crisis standards of care. The current report expands the focus to examine indicators and triggers across the entire continuum. This report describes indicators for all transitions along the continuum. It also uses the term *crisis care trigger* to describe triggers for the transition from contingency to crisis, and the term *trigger* to describe triggers at other boundaries along the continuum. Figure 1-1 has been updated to reflect this expanded focus.

[6] The format of the 2012 report was designed to reflect its purpose of providing a resource manual for all stakeholders involved in a disaster response. The first volume describes the overall framework and legal issues, and discusses the crosscutting themes of ethics, palliative care, and mental health. The next four volumes are each aimed at a key stakeholder group: state and local governments, EMS, hospitals and acute care facilities, and out-of-hospital and alternate care sites. Lastly, there is a volume on public engagement.

[7] The framework provides the overall systems approach; tactical-level responses are not included in Figure 1-2.

Incident demand/resource imbalance increases ────────────▶
Risk of morbidity/mortality to patient increases ────────────▶

Recovery ◀────────────

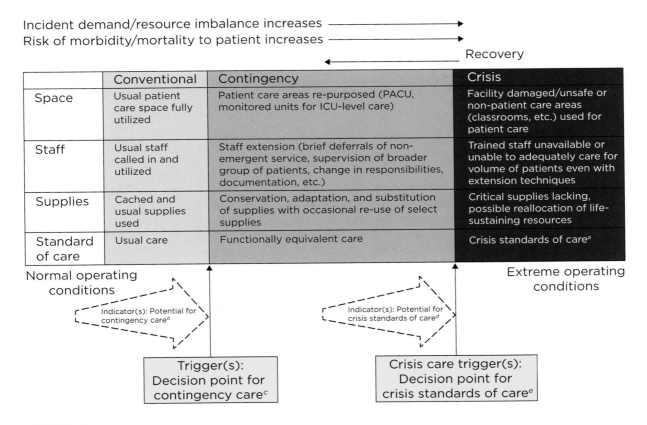

	Conventional	Contingency	Crisis
Space	Usual patient care space fully utilized	Patient care areas re-purposed (PACU, monitored units for ICU-level care)	Facility damaged/unsafe or non-patient care areas (classrooms, etc.) used for patient care
Staff	Usual staff called in and utilized	Staff extension (brief deferrals of non-emergent service, supervision of broader group of patients, change in responsibilities, documentation, etc.)	Trained staff unavailable or unable to adequately care for volume of patients even with extension techniques
Supplies	Cached and usual supplies used	Conservation, adaptation, and substitution of supplies with occasional re-use of select supplies	Critical supplies lacking, possible reallocation of life-sustaining resources
Standard of care	Usual care	Functionally equivalent care	Crisis standards of care[a]

Normal operating conditions

Extreme operating conditions

Indicator(s): Potential for contingency care[b]

Indicator(s): Potential for crisis standards of care[d]

Trigger(s): Decision point for contingency care[c]

Crisis care trigger(s): Decision point for crisis standards of care[e]

FIGURE 1-1
Allocation of specific resources along the care capacity continuum.
NOTE: ICU = intensive care unit; PACU = postanesthesia care unit. For clarity, the figure focuses on indicators and triggers for the transitions from conventional to contingency to crisis; it is also important to consider indicators and triggers that guide the return to conventional care.
[a] Unless temporary, requires state empowerment, clinical guidance, and protection for triage decisions and authorization for alternate care sites/techniques. Once situational awareness is achieved, triage decisions should be as systematic and well integrated into institutional process, review, and documentation as possible.
[b] Institutions may consider additional monitoring, analysis, and information sharing, and may prepare to implement select adaptive strategies (e.g., conserving resources where possible).
[c] Institutions implement select adaptive strategies and should consider impact on the community of resource use (i.e., consider "greatest good" vs. individual patient needs), but patient-centered decision making is still the focus.
[d] Institutions continue to implement select adaptive strategies, but also may need to prepare to make triage decisions and shift to community-centered decision making.
[e] Institutions (and providers) must make triage decisions—balancing the availability of resources to others and the individual patient needs—and shift to community-centered decision making.
SOURCE: Adapted from IOM, 2009, p. 53.

aspects of disaster planning and response to ensure that the needs of the community are met and the response is fair, just, and equitable. The 2009 report discusses the duty to plan by noting that "in an important ethical sense, entering a crisis standard of care mode is not optional—it is a forced choice, based on the emerging situation. Under such circumstances, failing to make substantive adjustments to care operations—i.e., not to adopt crisis standards of care—is very likely to result in greater death, injury, or illness" (IOM, 2009, p. 15). The other foundational element of the framework is the legal authority and environment that support the necessary and appropriate actions during a disaster response. Detailed consideration of legal issues is outside of the scope of this project, but issues related to legal indicators and triggers are raised briefly in Chapter 2 and examples are given in Chapter 5, the public health portion of the toolkit. For additional discussion and

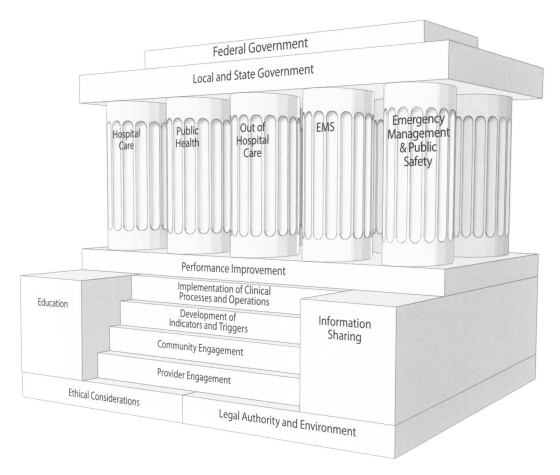

FIGURE 1-2
A systems framework for catastrophic disaster response.
NOTE: Ethical considerations and legal authority and environment form the foundation that undergirds crisis standards of care (CSC) planning and implementation. The steps represent key elements needed to implement disaster response. Education and information sharing are the cornerstones of the framework; together with the process of performance improvement, they support the key elements of CSC planning and enable midcourse corrections during the implementation of the framework. The response functions are performed by each of the five components of the emergency response system: hospitals and acute care, public health, out-of-hospital care, prehospital and emergency medical services (EMS), and emergency management/public safety. These components are interdependent in their contribution to the structure; they are joined by the roof, representing the overarching authority, additional resources, and protections offered by local, state, and federal governments.
SOURCE: IOM, 2012, p. 1-32.

details about the ethical and legal foundation, and other components of the framework described below, see the 2009 and 2012 reports.

The development of indicators and triggers was identified as a key step in the development of CSC plans (IOM, 2012). Following the release of the 2012 report, the development of indicators and triggers was specifically noted in the Hospital Preparedness Program and Public Health Emergency Preparedness cooperative agreements (ASPR, 2012a; CDC, 2011). The 2012 report contains extensive details about the roles and responsibilities for each component of the emergency response system, along with templates that identify core functions and tasks in both the planning and implementation of CSC. These templates use the same structure as the PHEP and HPP capabilities.

The emergency response system framework described above is consistent with the approach being encouraged by most local, state, and federal government agencies. Communities across the country are increasingly working to integrate and coordinate multiple emergency response disciplines under a single planning and response approach. FEMA, the federal agency chiefly responsible for coordinating crisis and consequence management, has emphasized a "whole of community" approach to catastrophic disaster planning (FEMA, 2011). The Department of Homeland Security (DHS) Office of Health Affairs and ASPR have collaborated on multiple efforts, ranging from chemical terrorism response to improving community resiliency (Cibulsky and Kirk, 2010; DHS, 2011). Along with DHS and ASPR, CDC, the Food and Drug Administration, the National Institutes of Health, the Department of Defense, the VA, and the Department of Agriculture are working together to explore the advances of medical countermeasures for use in biodefense, chemical response, and radiological emergencies, led by the Biomedical Advanced Research and Development Authority (BARDA) (ASPR, 2013a). These attempts demonstrate the importance of multiagency and multidisciplinary involvement in planning for the complex and challenging environment of large-scale disaster response.

The next two sections briefly discuss the roles of emergency management and state and local governments in developing and implementing CSC plans and, in particular, in facilitating information sharing. A discussion of the roles of VA Medical Centers and Military Treatment Facilities, including the use of indicators and triggers in these facilities, is included in Chapter 2.

Emergency Management

Because the successful implementation of CSC efforts requires full mobilization and participation of the entire emergency response system, local and state offices of emergency management can play an important role in serving as the conveners of subject matter experts and stakeholders responsible for the development of CSC plans. The 2012 report includes emergency management as a key component of the emergency response system, but the concepts presented in this section provide additional details beyond those included in that report. Table 1-1 summarizes the ways in which Emergency Support Functions (ESFs) work together to support public health and medical response, with emergency management providing coordination of these efforts.

The supportive efforts of emergency management, focused on the integration of the emergency response functions, begin with their role in running local (home ruled), regional, and/or state emergency operations centers (EOCs) and Multiagency Coordination Systems, and extend to the information that is exchanged under the auspices of such efforts. Some of this information may be specified by public health or state regulatory requirements, for example, the reporting of select infectious disease outbreaks that may have implications for the larger community, including those that may herald the onset of a bioterrorism attack. Other agencies, such as those involved in the delivery of out-of-hospital care, including mental health services and EMS agencies, may need to share important information that would be protected under the Health Insurance Portability and Accountability Act (HIPAA) outside an emergency situation. Such information is sometimes not shared on account of uncertainties pertaining to the range and applicability of these existing regulations. Sharing clinical data, particularly deidentified data, can be an important adjunct to the creation of real-time awareness needed to help inform decision makers, particularly during epidemics. This is where

TABLE 1-1
Roles and Responsibilities of the Emergency Support Functions (ESFs)

	Examples of the Ways in Which ESFs Work Together to Support Public Health and Medical Response, with Emergency Management Providing Coordination of These Efforts
ESF-1 – Transportation	Aviation/airspace management and control • Coordinate landing zone location for air medical transport (helicopter and fixed wing) operations • Request "no-fly" zones from the Federal Aviation Administration (FAA) as required to provide safe air medical and ground operational environments Transportation safety • Damage and impact assessment • Coordinate establishment of transportation corridors for use by ground emergency medical services (EMS) transport units, logistics support for supplies, evacuation needs of population • Assist with identification of alternate casualty transport mechanisms if needed, such as school buses, large transport vehicles accessible to wheelchair users, aircraft or watercraft, etc. Restoration/recovery of transportation infrastructure Aquatic/waterfront management and control • Coordinate sites for patient transfers between water rescue and dive teams and ground EMS and air medical teams • Provide logistics support for transfer and transport of supplies and equipment to waterborne rescue and medical teams
ESF-2 – Communications	Restoration and repair of communications infrastructure • Assure communications support to health care organizations, 911 call centers Coordinate communications among local, state, and federal incident management and response structures
ESF-3 – Public Works and Engineering	Infrastructure protection, emergency repair and restoration • Preidentify hospitals and health care organizations for priority utility service restoration • Prioritize health care facilities for service support during an incident (road access, generators, etc.) Provide contracting support for life-saving and life-sustaining services needed during an incident or [a] planned event
ESF-4 – Firefighting	Provide support to wildland, rural, and urban firefighting operations • Assure mitigation and risk reduction strategies related to fire safety are in place for disaster-affected health care facilities
ESF-5 – Emergency Management	Coordination of incident management and response efforts across entire event (short term or sustained) • Ensure ESF-8 needs are appropriately prioritized and adequately resourced • Assist in coordination of resource and human capital to support ESF-8 requirements • Provide leadership and direction for incident action planning that occurs within ESF-8 • Establish processes and procedures to ensure appropriate financial management and recovery of costs • Support facilities, security, and logistics if needed for alternate care sites, and distribution and dispensing nodes for public health and medical equipment and supplies
ESF-6 – Mass Care, Emergency Assistance, Housing, and Human Services	Support the ability and maintain the lead role to provide mass care and sheltering • Facilitate planning with local health departments and health care organizations on shelter operations planning and response, including medical special needs shelters • Coordinate with health care organizations in conjunction with public health to assure that medical needs are being met for sheltered population • Coordinate with public health and health care organizations to assure that the reunification of families and households is facilitated by patient tracking mechanisms and occupant logs of shelters
ESF-7 – Logistics Management and Resource Support	Provide incident logistics planning, management, and sustainment capability • Provide resource support (supplies, contracting services, etc.), including provision of water, sanitation, and backup electrical services to affected health care organizations • Provide support to alleviate identified supply chain issues related to public health and medical

CRISIS STANDARDS OF CARE: A TOOLKIT FOR INDICATORS AND TRIGGERS

TABLE 1-1
Continued

	Examples of the Ways in Which ESFs Work Together to Support Public Health and Medical Response, with Emergency Management Providing Coordination of These Efforts
ESF-8 – Public Health and Medical Services	Ensure coordination of health and medical response in these specific areas (see remainder of Table 1-1): • Public health • Medical, including EMS • Mental health services • Mass fatality management • Veterinary medical support
ESF-9 – Search and Rescue	Search and rescue operations • Facilitate coordination between local emergency response agencies and receiving health care facilities that will provide medical care to ill and injured
ESF-10 – Oil and Hazardous Materials Response	Hazardous materials (chemical, biological, radiological, etc.) response • Coordinate response needs with public health, EMS, and health care organizations to assure consistent approach to use of personal protective equipment and need for medical countermeasures • Provide decontamination support and washwater containment support for victim decontamination operations as requested by public safety agencies/health care facilities • Ensure establishment of perimeters when appropriate based on sampling or modeling Environmental short- and long-term cleanup • Proactively engage ESF-8 partners in mitigating any potential foreseen or unforeseen medical concerns related to contamination events • Support epidemiological studies of the health impacts of environmental contamination
ESF-11 – Agriculture and Natural Resources	Provide for animal welfare needs, coordination of response to plant disease and pest response • Assure support (access to veterinary care, food) available for service animals Coordinate food safety and security oversight requirements Provide for safety and well-being of household pets per local plans Coordinate management of mass fatalities of animals
ESF-12 – Energy	Energy infrastructure assessment, repair, and restoration • Assure priority restoration of services to impacted health care organizations • Facilitate the provision of fuel for generators, etc., as required at health care facilities and for ground, air, and waterborne emergency response organizations • Support monitoring and possible decontamination for radiological emergencies
ESF-13 – Public Safety and Security	Ensure access to public safety and security support • Prioritize health care facility and resource security • Provide support to access, traffic, and crowd control that may affect health care organizations in the immediate aftermath of a disaster event • Coordinate access by health care providers to "secured" areas to enable staffing of hospitals • Provide security for transportation and administration of community-based interventions (distribution of countermeasures, vaccine, etc.)
ESF-14 – Long-Term Community Recovery	Social and economic community impact assessment Long-term community recovery assistance to states, local governments, and the private sector to restore damaged health care facilities Analysis and review of mitigation program implementation to prevent future damage to health care organizations (e.g., moving generators to roofs in flood-prone areas) Stress management and personal resilience resources assessment for public health and medical staff Analysis and review of repatriation of families and households that require home care (e.g., home ventilator patients)
ESF-15 – External Affairs	Emergency public information and protective action guidance • Coordinate participation of ESF-8 partners in Joint Information System planning and response • Provide health messages relevant to the event to targeted populations Assist in coordination of media and community relations

SOURCE: Adapted from FEMA, 2008b.

public health should work with emergency management to ensure that appropriate data are shared to the level needed for response.

Information crucial to the monitoring of key indicators governing the change in delivery of health care services is likely to be most easily gathered, analyzed, and shared through the EOC during an incident. Given the usual functioning of EOCs, this is the single physical location where representatives from across the emergency response system are co-located, further facilitating the exchange of key information and the request for desired resources. In a sustained health incident, emergency management may still need to be connected to the remainder of the components of the emergency response system. It is possible to create a "virtual" EOC connection, particularly useful for slow-onset or sustained incidents such as an influenza pandemic, in which the monitoring function will persist for weeks or months. The need to staff a "physical location," in this example, is less important than having the connectivity to share information with the emergency response community over the period of time that the response conditions are affected by the incident.

Emergency management agencies can help broker efforts to coordinate and analyze a variety of information sources, including from utilities and private enterprise, in the context of large-scale disaster incidents that will be marked by many different data feeds; sources of information, including the use of social media inputs; and the need to "roll up" information to make it usable and actionable. It is understood that the State Public Health Emergency Coordination Center[8] would play a critical role in working with emergency management, particularly as it relates to the indicators and triggers being evaluated for CSC implementation, as further elaborated below.

State and Local Governments

State and local governments play a critical role in collecting information and providing access to such information on a day-to-day basis as well as during times of crisis. Specific to the planning efforts required for crisis standards of care implementation, state and local governments—but particularly the state departments of health (with active engagement of state EMS offices and prehospital care agencies)—will be key conveners of the CSC stakeholders, and will help to develop the protocols and identify the areas of greatest interest pertaining to data flow and information exchange. The 2009 and 2012 reports provided extensive discussion of the roles of state and local governments, with a particular focus on state and local departments of health (or other most relevant entity, depending on the state/local structure), in planning and implementing CSC (IOM, 2009, 2012).

The Medical Surge Capacity and Capability (MSCC) framework outlines a tiered system of relationships among individual health care organizations, health care coalitions, and local, state, and federal governments (Barbera and Macintyre, 2007, 2009). Figure 1-3 shows the integration of CSC planning and response into the MSCC framework, including specific entities that develop and help implement CSC, such as state and regional disaster medical advisory committees (or equivalent), triage teams, clinical care committees, and palliative care teams. For additional information about the roles of these entities, see Table 2-2 in the 2012 report, as well as the 2009 report (IOM, 2009, 2012).

Integrated planning within and across tiers is critical for a coordinated response, as all entities should

---

[8] Depending on the state, this may be referred to in a variety of ways, including state (public) health emergency coordination center, department of (public) health operation center, or state (public) health operation center.

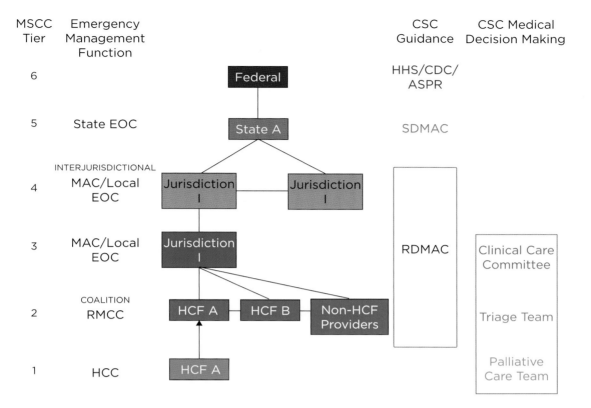

FIGURE 1-3
Integrating crisis standards of care planning into the Medical Surge Capacity and Capability framework.
NOTES: See Table 2-2 in IOM (2012) for further detail and description of the functions of these entities. The clinical care committee, triage team, and palliative care team may be established at MSCC tiers 1, 2, or 3. The RDMAC may be established at MSCC tiers 2, 3, or 4, depending on local agreements. The RMCC is linked to the MAC/Local EOC and is intended to provide regional health and medical information in those communities; it functions at MSCC tiers 2-4. ASPR = Assistant Secretary for Preparedness and Response (Department of Health and Human Services); CDC = Centers for Disease Control and Prevention; CSC = crisis standards of care; EOC = emergency operations center; HCC = health care coalition; HCF = health care facility; HHS = Department of Health and Human Services; MAC = Medical Advisory Committee; RDMAC = Regional Disaster Medical Advisory Committee; RMCC = Regional Medical Coordination Center; SDMAC = State Disaster Medical Advisory Committee.
SOURCE: Adapted from IOM, 2012, p. 1-44.

understand the situation of the other entities before moving to a different level of response along the continuum of care. As a disaster unfolds, the facilitation of access to additional vetted information will likely come from federal, state, tribal, and local government authorities. But this will happen only if preincident planning regarding the approach to CSC implementation has taken place. Otherwise, access to information is likely to be ad hoc and may obscure a complete assessment of the situation at hand. State and local governments are the most important entities in helping to support such planning. They serve as the conduit from agencies and health care organizations at the local level to state-level authorities, as well as from the state to their respective federal partners. Horizontal and vertical integration (within and across tiers) of the planning effort is critical to the success of CSC planning, particularly as it relates to achieving situational awareness based on preidentified indicators of the transition from conventional surge response toward contingency and crisis response. The data points being evaluated in one corner of the state, resulting in decisions taken regarding the access to potentially scarce resources and the delivery of care, should be the same as those being reviewed and acted on in other areas of the state or adjoining states. Not to do so, or to plan for such coordination, goes against one of the fundamental recommendations of the IOM CSC effort, namely, the importance of achieving intrastate and interstate coordination (IOM, 2009). Instead of using the MSCC framework and creating another response framework, some states may have existing regional and state infrastructures for inclusive trauma/EMS advisory councils/committees; the points made above about the importance of including all response partners and ensuring horizontal and vertical integration within and across tiers apply equally regardless of the specific framework used.

In addition to responders at the state, local, health care coalition, and health care organization levels, other responders may come from federal National Disaster Medical System (NDMS) teams (ASPR, 2012b). Box 1-3 explores the role of NDMS responders, including disaster medical assistance teams.

BOX 1-3
Role of National Disaster Medical System (NDMS) Responders

Large-scale disaster incidents that require the use of federal resources, including the deployment of NDMS response teams, are likely to be the types of incidents in which the delivery of care may shift, at some point, across the conventional to contingency to crisis surge response continuum. NDMS is composed of four types of teams: Disaster Medical Assistance Team (DMAT), Disaster Mortuary Operational Response Team (DMORT), International Medical Surgical Response Team (IMSURT), and National Veterinary Response Team (NVRT). It is incumbent on federal responders, including those who comprise the NDMS response teams, to understand the context in which they are being asked to deliver health and medical services. Under disaster response conditions, it is likely that the care being delivered falls in the categories of contingency (functionally equivalent) or even crisis care. Establishing tent-based or alternate care site response capabilities in hospital parking lots, for example, can never equate to the degree of care offered in an intact health care facility. Yet, it can provide functionally equivalent care, using a no-frills approach to basic medical care delivery. Under more catastrophic conditions, where only select patient care needs can be met under such circumstances, it is likely that more sophisticated diagnostic capabilities and treatment options are simply not going to be available. Surgical services provided under "battlefield" conditions would be examples by which the federal response teams are providing care under crisis standards. Having to do so, in and of itself, is suggestive of a community-wide "indicator" that the health care infrastructure remains disrupted, save for the establishment and use of these federal resources. Diagnostic capabilities, treatment modalities, documentation of services, and even the types and levels of providers who attend to specific medical needs may all be significantly different than what would be the conventional approach to health care needs in the non-affected state.

Lessons from Hurricane Katrina and the Port au Prince Earthquake

An exploration of the ethical underpinnings related to catastrophic disaster response is an important adjunct to the preparation of health care professionals who take on the responsibilities of joining the NDMS response system. This includes understanding the criteria related to scarce resource allocation, as well as the processes by which triage decisions are taken. Deciding who gets what level of care, when not all patients can be treated equally, are some of the hard lessons learned from the response of NDMS teams to Hurricane Katrina and the Haiti earthquake (Klein et al., 2008; Merin et al., 2010). Are resources that are available to the NDMS responders adequate to meet patient needs? Would their application to few patients potentially compromise their ability to provide

---

Indicators and Triggers in the PHEP and HPP Capabilities and in the Overall CSC Planning Process

Both the CDC PHEP and the ASPR HPP cooperative agreements specifically call for the development of CSC plans, including indicators (ASPR, 2012a, 2013b; CDC, 2011). Completion of the tables in this toolkit will help users develop appropriate protocol and plans in accordance with the national guidance set forth in the HPP and PHEP documents. Box 1-4 outlines the primary capabilities, functions, and plans that

care for many others who might benefit more? These and related questions are also important considerations in response to complex humanitarian emergencies outside of the United States, where the existing standards of care are fundamentally different from those at home, and the medical and cultural expectations are likely to be very different. It is particularly important to recognize that response to such incidents abroad must come with a longer commitment to support the recovery and rebuilding in the affected countries (Subbarao et al., 2010).

Response teams should coordinate their efforts with the local emergency management agencies, and ensure that as federal assets, they are coordinating the application of their resources in accordance with local needs. In addition, given the dynamic nature of such incidents, it is incumbent on response teams to maintain good communications in the disaster zone, as well as back to the command and control oversight teams that accompany their deployment. Given availability of resources and patient care requirements, it is clear that decisions taken one day, for example, with respect to categorization of patients by triage category, may change. The patients categorized in the "expectant" category during the operations conducted at the New Orleans Louis Armstrong Airport shifted over time as more resources became available and patients' conditions changed (Klein et al., 2008). Health care providers who are engaged in such missions must recognize the responsibilities that accompany these deployments, the nature of shifting conditions, and the manner by which they make these decisions, grounded in ethical considerations and the rule of law.

Response to Hurricane Sandy

In the week after the storm severely impacted the metropolitan New York and New Jersey region, causing the displacement of many hundreds of patients from hospitals and nursing homes that had to be evacuated due to rising flood waters and loss of electricity (Carcamo, 2012), the NDMS response was in full swing. Fourteen DMATS, two teams of U.S. Public Health Service commissioned corps officers, and seven Federal Medical Stations were deployed to the region. One of the Federal Medical Stations was established to serve as a medical shelter, in the attempts to keep patients from seeking care at already overburdened hospitals. The DMATs, with their caches of medical supplies and pharmaceuticals, were deployed across the metro region to provide care in established medical shelters and, in certain cases, to augment hospital staff (ASPR, 2012c). These resources allowed contingency care to be maintained in areas that otherwise might have been faced with a health care crisis situation due to the infrastructure damage.

are addressed by this toolkit. However, the discussions prompted by this toolkit cover a broader set of areas, including information sharing, partnership development, systems coordination, and medical surge planning. Therefore, Box 1-4 also lists other HPP and PHEP capabilities that will be augmented through the toolkit discussions.

As described in the 2012 report, the third step in the CSC planning process should be the identification of indicators and triggers. For communities that are in the early stages of the CSC planning process, the use

o Surge Assessment:
    ◆ Pre-incident assessment of normal operating capacity for healthcare organizations within the healthcare delivery area
    ◆ Pre-incident estimate of surge casualties (i.e., medical casualties, mental/behavioral health casualties)
    ◆ Pre-incident assessment of available resources to address surge estimates
    ◆ Development of surge capacity indicators that would trigger different aspects of the medical surge plan (e.g., surge in place strategies; early discharge, cancelled elective surgeries; augmented personnel; extra shifts, volunteers; established alternate care sites or activated mobile units; requested mutual aid)
    ◆ Processes to immediately identify an increase in medical surge status during an incident (e.g., medical, mental/behavioral health, concerned individuals)

Capability 10: Medical Surge, Function 4: Develop crisis standards of care guidance
  • Task 2: Identify the guidelines for crisis standards of care, including the effective allocation of scarce resources
  • Resource Elements: Plans (P)
    o P1: State crisis standards of care guidance
    o P2: Indicators for crisis standards of care
    o P3: Legal protections for healthcare practitioners and institutions
    o P4: Provide guidance for crisis standards of care implementation processes
    o P5: Provide guidance for the management of scarce resources

Other relevant capabilities:
Capability 1: Healthcare System Preparedness
Capability 3: Emergency Operations Coordination
Capability 6: Information Sharing

Hospital Preparedness Program (HPP) Measure Manual: Implementation Guidance for the HPP Program Measures (2013)

Capability Roadmap for Medical Surge
  • Indicator #1: The awardee has posted its approved crisis standards of care plan on the ASPR Communities of Interest SharePoint Site.

SOURCES: ASPR, 2012a, 2013b; CDC, 2011.

of this toolkit, and the exploration of community, regional, and state-derived indicators, triggers, and the process by which actions are then taken, would be an excellent place to start this important work.

The 2012 report also highlighted the "milestones" for CSC planning. The establishment of indicators and triggers most easily fits within the fourth milestone: *Developing a state health and medical approach to CSC planning that can be adopted at the regional/local level by existing health care coalitions, emergency response systems (including the Regional Disaster Medical Advisory Committee), and health care providers* (IOM, 2012, p. 1-5).

This suggests that the discussion of indicators and triggers should be started relatively early in the CSC planning process, particularly as it provides much of the needed detail about what it means to transition away from conventional response and toward the delivery of health care that occurs in the contingency arena, or in worst cases, under crisis conditions.

Specialized Surge Capabilities

Pediatric and burn mass casualty incidents are presented as examples that require planning for specific surge capabilities in order to ensure the best possible patient care outcomes. (Table 1-2 outlines considerations.)

TABLE 1-2
Surge Considerations for Pediatric and Burn Care

	Pediatric	Burn
Stabilization	Pediatric equipment, including guides for weight-based equipment selection and drug dosing (liquid medications), and appropriately trained providers must be available at *all* emergency departments to stabilize patients, with emphasis on those <8 years of age.	Basic dressings, analgesia, fluid support, and airway management should be available at *all* emergency departments. Providers should be trained in initial stabilization and management of burn victims in order to avoid critical errors in resuscitation.
Surge capacity	Specific spaces that are safe and appropriate for pediatric care must be identified, as well as the requisite equipment and staff with pediatric expertise necessary for appropriate care. Increased staffing ratios are required to safely care for children. Strategies for adaptation of equipment or medications in adults may not be applicable to the pediatric population. Specific support and safety issues must be addressed—a pediatric safe area, nutrition (including infant formula), psychological support, etc. Non-pediatric hospitals may have to provide inpatient care for pediatric patients during epidemic or mass casualty incidents.	Major burn patients require large amounts of intravenous fluids and narcotic analgesia. Burn unit beds are in critically short supply in the United States and in mass casualty incidents non-burn unit hospitals may have to manage burn victims for at least the first few days. Will need tiered triage to transport those most likely to benefit from care at a burn center over time.
Tracking	Reunification of children with their caregivers is a critical focus of pediatric planning. Policies and processes need to be in place prior to an incident. Information on transfers must be easily shared between organizations to facilitate this process.	Information on number of victims, condition, and transfers must be easily shared among organizations to facilitate appropriate transfers and reunification, especially when regional transfers are required.
Coordination	Incident demand must be balanced across coalition facilities that provide (or can provide) pediatric care and other networks of children's hospitals. Pediatric subject matter experts or pediatric health care coalitions should be integrated into the transfer framework to provide input on appropriate destinations and use of available beds for specific patients.	Incident demand must be balanced across coalition facilities that provide (or can provide) burn care and burn center networks. Subject matter experts should be integrated into the transfer framework to provide input on appropriate destinations and use of available beds for specific patients so debridement and interventions can be appropriately timed.
Consultation	Must be available for hospitals that have to manage pediatric patients that do not normally do so. Telemedicine, telephone, and other methods of consultation are imperative, and these may need to be set up with national pediatric centers or with pediatric health care coalitions if the local/regional centers of expertise are too overwhelmed to provide such support.	Must be available for hospitals that have to manage burn patients that do not normally do so. Telemedicine, telephone, and other methods of consultation are imperative—and these may need to be set up with national burn centers if the local/regional centers of expertise are too overwhelmed to provide such support.
Transportation	Pediatric patients may have specific transport needs (bassinets, car seats, other safety restraints, appropriate pediatric-sized equipment for en-route care, e.g., IV pumps).	Burn patients need to be protected against hypothermia during transport, and adequate analgesia, fluids, and airway equipment are required for safe transfer.

In each case—managing pediatric patients or managing burn patients—specific resources, including knowledgeable and experienced health care providers, may not be readily available to provide care. However, planning for common approaches to regional training and response frameworks may be used to meet the needs of very different incidents (for additional consideration, see, for example, Appendix D in IOM, 2012, which outlines resource challenges by disaster type, and NCIPC, 2007, which discusses surge capacity for a terrorist bombing).

Resource shortages associated with specialized capabilities, such as pediatric and burn care, are more likely to occur in a non-catastrophic incident. Higher tiers in the MSCC framework may have to be activated for lower numbers of victims, compared to nonspecialized capabilities (Barbera and Macintyre, 2007, 2009). These types of examples may, therefore, provide insight into how care changes and how transitions across the continuum of care should be considered, as every health care facility must plan to initially receive these types of patients (see AAP et al., 2009, and Kearns, 2011).

IMPLEMENTATION OF THE DISASTER RESPONSE FRAMEWORK

The 2012 report outlines a process for decision making during a disaster, providing a systems approach to help health care organizations determine whether health care delivery can remain at the conventional level, or whether contingency and/or crisis care should be implemented (see Figure 1-4). The "planning A" cycle is based on the well-honed concept used as part of an emergency management system known as the "planning P" (FEMA, 2008a). This is a combination of management by objectives that relies on the development of specific strategies and the tactics needed to support those strategies, with a time phase element included to ensure that progress and improvements in the response to any given incident are being noted, and when they are not, allows for midcourse adjustments and a shift in strategies and tactics. This would occur within the context of an incident command system that is compatible with the National Incident Management System (NIMS), such as the Hospital Incident Command System (HICS) (EMSA, 2007; FEMA, 2013).

This graphical depiction highlights the dynamic qualities of any given incident, regardless of whether it is one that develops slowly over time, or a sudden onset, no-notice incident. The transition from conventional to contingency response occurs with the crossing of the resource shortage threshold. A shortage in any given resource—both material and personnel items (supplies, equipment, pharmaceuticals) and humans (health care providers)—may result in this threshold being crossed. At this point, strategies and tactics can be employed to attempt to move back toward the delivery of care under conventional conditions. These strategies include conservation, substitution, adaptation, and even reuse of certain resources.[9]

At some point, however, with severe and sustained shortages of key resources, the ability to deliver medical care services under contingency conditions will be compromised. The goal should be for these adaptations to move care back toward conventional. However, if the situation worsens, extension of these adaptive strategies may be required. At this point, the strategies of conservation, substitution, adaptation, and reuse of resources are extended to the point that they no longer ensure functionally equivalent care.

---

[9] A recent comparative effectiveness review of strategies for managing and allocating resources during mass casualty incidents categorizes strategies as follows: reduce or manage less urgent demand for health care services, optimize use of existing resources, augment existing resources, and crisis standards of care (Timbie et al., 2012, 2013).

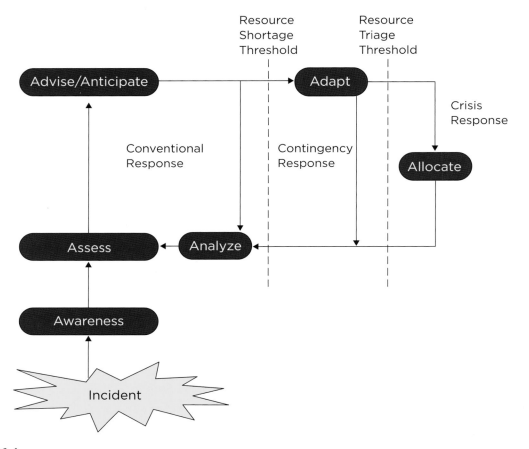

FIGURE 1-4
Implementation of the Surge Response Framework: Conventional, contingency, and crisis response cycle.
After an incident occurs, the first priority is to develop situational **Awareness**, and then to **Assess** the situation relative to the available resources. The incident commander, along with relevant technical experts and/or the clinical care committee (in a proactive response/longer-term incident) **Advises** on strategies and **Anticipates** any resource deficits (and recommends obtaining necessary supplies, staffing, etc.). If a resource is scarce, **Adaptive** strategies (e.g., conservation, substitution, adaptation, and reuse) should be implemented. In a crisis, a deliberate triage decision to **Allocate**/reallocate resources may be necessary. In all cases, the response and any strategies should be **Analyzed** at regular intervals as part of the disaster response planning cycle, and the elements repeated until the incident concludes.
SOURCE: IOM, 2012, p. 1-48.

Supplies, space, and staff have to be employed in a way that presents a risk of a compromised outcome to the patient. Thus, contingency and crisis care may coexist in this area depending on the degree to which the strategies are extended.

Lack of specific treatment resources may require that a health care organization also cross the resource triage threshold. Under these conditions, there are not enough resources available relative to the demand for care, and key resources must be triaged for patients. Reallocation of scarce resources will be needed, based on population-based values (derived from community engagement inputs) and population-based outcomes (based on what limited evidence base may be available to support such decisions) and is inherently located in the crisis portion of the continuum.

In general the space before reaching a *resource shortage threshold* corresponds to *conventional* care, the space after crossing that threshold but before reaching the *resource triage threshold* corresponds to *contingency* care, and the space after crossing the *resource triage threshold* corresponds to *crisis* care. However, the discussion above makes clear that there are gray areas in the *resource shortage* space, where a combination of contingency and crisis care may be delivered depending on the resources that are scarce and the strategies that are being implemented. For example, depending on the resource that is being reused, the care may be considered functionally equivalent or it may present a risk to patient outcomes. The extent to which staff members are practicing within or beyond their usual or comfortable scope of practice and supervision is another example.

This indicators and triggers toolkit is intended to expand on the concepts described above, including issues such as sources of indicator information, types of triggers and decision making, and what information planners and decision makers can use to make these determinations. These questions are particularly challenging given the dynamic conditions during such incidents, the number of resources and other variables involved in providing care, and the many different potential resource shortages that could occur during the response.

THE NEED TO DEVELOP INDICATORS AND TRIGGERS

The need for the development of indicators and triggers for crisis standards of care has been discussed in a number of studies and reports throughout the past 5 years (Devereaux et al., 2008; IOM, 2009, 2012; Joynt et al., 2010). Recommendations to define and incorporate clear indicators and triggers into preparedness protocols were highlighted in the two IOM reports (IOM, 2009, 2012). Developing indicators and triggers at all levels of the emergency response system, as outlined in Figure 1-2, will help ensure consistency in the implementation of CSC. The identification of specific measurements and predictors throughout the planning process is critical to determining appropriate actions and decision making. In addition, the development and use of indicators and triggers can help support responders' behavioral health and resilience.

Individuals involved in disaster response should understand what sources of information are available to inform decision making, what authorities they have, and what the plan is for pulling the trigger—who will do it, how, and when. This type of planning needs to be done in advance to allow the necessary dialogue about sources of information, integration, authorities, and processes.

Experience, training, information sharing, and data interpretation are key factors that influence decision making during crises, particularly given the impact of stress, complexity, uncertainty, and time pressure associated with such situations (see Box 1-5). The careful monitoring of indicators is likely an important determinant of successful incident response. As noted by Alberts (2007, p. 19), "focus represents a synthesis of how [a] situation is perceived and understood, including perceptions about the nature of the endeavor (strategies and plans) that are appropriate for the situation." In the context of crisis response, there should be a focus on the indicators that are used to determine that a transition in care is occurring across the surge continuum. Leaders and decision makers involved in having to make scarce resource allocation decisions require reliable, authenticated, predictive, and actionable data on which they will make important choices during a crisis incident. The development of indicators and triggers can also provide a standard operating procedure for line employees to rely on, although this is only appropriate for certain types of information and decisions, as will be discussed in Chapter 2.

Box 1-6 discusses issues related to the decision to evacuate health care facilities or shelter in place. This decision illustrates the difficulty of decisions made during disasters and the importance of advance planning.

BOX 1-5
Decision Making in Crises

Making reasoned decisions in a stressful situation is one of the most important skills for a first responder. This is true for those in leadership roles such as the incident commander, those managing the National Incident Management System (NIMS) designed response hierarchy support functions, field-based uniformed-services first responders, health professionals, and nontraditional emergency responders. Facing unique and dynamic situational environments and the psychological pressure of adapting well-practiced work routines into novel response sets is very challenging. The adverse impact of personal stress on decision making is well documented.

The literature on decision making associated with crisis situations consistently identifies stress and fatigue as contributing factors having a detrimental effect on the decision-making process (Brecher, 1979; Helmreich and Merritt, 1998; Rosenthal and t'Hart, 1991). Stress primarily has been shown to negatively affect decision making (Keinan, 1987; Kowalski-Trakofler and Vaught, 2003; Staal, 2004). In particular, people consider fewer alternatives and options, rely on prior decisions made in similar situations (even when ineffective), and have the potential to reach an overall state of attentional disorganization. Similar findings were also seen when decisions had to be made within pressing time constraints (Zakay, 1993). In addition, uncertainty and lack of information can lead to misguided and suboptimal decision making (Bell, 1982; Hansson, 1996; Sarter and Schroeder, 2001).

As an incident progresses, the quality of decision making at all leadership and responder levels is threatened. Renaud (2012) recently suggested a straightforward cognitive approach for thinking through chaotic situations before deciding on an action. She suggests a cognitive strategy for accessing the situational demands of the incident, comparing the current event to past experience, identifying what one needs to know, what one does not know, and ultimately what one wants, and can and must do. All of this should occur within the context of the assigned mission goals of what must be accomplished. This process helps keep decision making relevant to the current incident, and decision makers from rushing too quickly to judgment and action based on excessive reliance on past experience.

Extreme events (catastrophic) and adaptive decision making also involves monitoring of the response environment and the changing capabilities of responders to competently carry out their duties over time. Other data (Burkle and Hayden, 2001) on emergency response decision making indicate that decision making in isolation is not effective in managing unique and rapidly changing large-scale disaster events. Abandoning vertical or stovepipe organizational models for lateral management models improves communication and data acquisition necessary for dynamic decision making. Decision-making capabilities during a large-scale incident are enhanced though preplanning strategies, practicing response plans, and building a response framework that recognizes threats to responder health and sustained response capabilities by integrating responder physical and psychological health care strategies into response protocols (HHS, 2005).

Crew resource management (CRM) training, principles of human factors, and the use of checklists are also valuable resources to potentially enhance decision making in disasters. CRM was developed as a training resource to decrease error through the use of behavioral countermeasures that address human factors that can lead to error. Recognizing the influence of stress, fatigue, and other situational and individual factors on cognitive processes (WHO, 2009), CRM is not meant to eliminate human error, but rather to encourage appropriate error management and safety (Helmreich et al., 1999). Strategies to promote teamwork, communication, situational awareness, interpersonal skills, leadership, and decision making are addressed in this predominantly simulation-based training (Flin et al., 2002). The use of checklists has also been discussed in great detail, particularly in aviation and more recently in the medical context, as a means to inform and guide decision making. Checklists, when used properly, can manage error, reduce risk, increase patient safety, and serve as quality control (Walker et al., 2012; Winters et al., 2009). However, each of these resources has limitations that must be considered. Findings from several studies revealed predominantly positive results regarding the effectiveness of CRM on attitudes, reactions, and learning, yet mixed results on behavior (O'Connor et al., 2008; Salas et al., 2006). Although checklists have been found to be beneficial tools, it is important to note that they must be considered within the context of the overall system; the environment, technology, and human error can ultimately influence outcomes (Degani and Wiener, 1993; Mauro et al., 2012). Therefore, it is particularly important for decision makers to consider additional approaches and strategies based on the situation at hand.

Key points: Stress adversely impacts decision making at all levels; there are strategies that can help enhance decision making; planning and practicing facilitates better decisions as long as this does not cause decision makers to reduce the ability to consider novel and innovative approaches.

BOX 1-6
Making the Decision: Evacuation Versus Shelter in Place

Given the complexities involved in conducting partial and full-scale health care facility evacuations, particularly under the duress of an emergency incident, both the decision taken "to stay" and the calculus applied "to go" is fraught with risk. Choosing to move patients and staff ahead of an impending storm can be a very difficult maneuver to execute, may result in increased morbidity and mortality to patients, and introduces a heightened risk associated with the movement of patients, whether by air or ground transportation. In 2005, 23 nursing home patients were killed in a bus fire after being evacuated from a facility in Houston in preparation for the arrival of Hurricane Rita (NTSB, 2007). When it arrived, Houston was spared the brunt of the storm's effects. On the other hand, choosing to shelter patients and staff in place, to hunker down and let the storm pass or conditions stabilize, may be equally risky, as evidenced most recently by the infrastructure failures in two lower Manhattan hospitals during Hurricane Sandy, prompting spontaneous decisions to evacuate at the height of the storm, and soon thereafter (Fink, 2012). It could be said, then, that the decisions taken around whether to evacuate versus sheltering in place can amount to no better than a Pyrrhic victory.

The decision-making process to either shelter in place or evacuate a health care facility in response to a disaster incident, both sudden onset (earthquake) and anticipated (hurricane), requires assessing a number of interrelated variables and determining the risk related to each one taken independently, and then together (Downey et al., 2013a,b; Sexton et al., 2007; Sternberg et al., 2004; Zaenger et al., 2010):

- Impact: How much time is available to make a decision? How severe is the storm expected to be? What is its projected path? Will critical utilities or access to the facility likely be compromised? If a decision to evacuate is deferred, will a later decision to evacuate carry an increased safety risk?
- Infrastructure: Does the health care facility have specific vulnerabilities related to infrastructure support and storm resiliency? Are there sufficient staffing and resources to support extended operations under duress? Are alternate locations available to send patients? Are means available to get patients out of harm's way, if necessary? Are there any plans by the utilities to cut power or gas supply to the impacted area after the storm to prevent injury and fires?
- Incident specific: Preparedness efforts must take into account the known variables, as well as the rapid assessment and integration of event-specific variables that develop during the incident, and must be flexible enough to be able to adapt to changing circumstances. These may include the ability of emergency medical services (EMS) to support evacuation operations, and other community and facility factors. Radiation and the presence of hazardous materials also impacts decision making.

In July 2006, the Government Accountability Office report on this issue found that hospitals and nursing home facility administrative leaders noted that they considered evacuation a decision of "last resort," and that their emergency plans were primarily designed to shelter in place (GAO, 2006). Moreover, it highlighted the issue that despite some jurisdictional calls for "mandatory evacuation," some health care organizations may not be capable of complying with the requested actions given the lack of suitable transportation and the staff to accompany patients. At the same time, few hospitals would choose to evacuate on their own, without a formal governmental recommendation/order to do so due to the anticipated impact on business operations (Schultz et al., 2003). Making matters worse, the loss of communications infrastructure can significantly impede decision making in real time, as conditions change and a stay-or-go decision must be made. Despite health care organization accreditation processes that include written plans for evacuation, this is a skill that is rarely, if ever, tested given the logistical challenges faced with doing so, and the exorbitant expense that would be incurred to take on a full-scale exercise (see Femino et al., 2013; Jen et al., 2009).

Once a commitment is made to evacuate, immediate follow-on decisions are required (Zane et al., 2010):

- Is the evacuation to be partial or complete? Plans must be made to ensure the scalability of these efforts, recognizing that conditions resulting in the movement of some patients may ultimately require the evacuation of all patients. A subset of high-technology dependent patients (e.g., ventilator dependent, intra-aortic balloon pump) may be at such elevated risk from a move that unless the facility clearly cannot continue operations, a shelter-in-place strategy may be most appropriate for them.
- If a partial evacuation is warranted, should remaining patients be moved to more accessible areas of the hospital, in order to facilitate their rapid evacuation, should the necessity arise based on changing conditions?
- Are the most critically ill, resource-dependent patients triaged to be moved first, or are they the last to be moved?
- In the absence of specialized equipment used to help facilitate the evacuation of patients, can an evacuation plan still be carried out?
- How are destination hospitals selected and how is acceptance of patients arranged?
- What staging areas and evacuation process will be used (designated stairwells vs. elevators, mechanisms of movement, etc.)?
- What paperwork/chart information will be sent with the patients?
- What transportation resources are available, and in what time frame? Will they continue to be available as the event continues/progresses?

Many of these secondary decisions can be managed in stepwise fashion, but in all cases, the decision makers will have to convey expectations to the patient units (except in the case of a catastrophic impact on the facility when each unit must recognize the immediate safety risk and proceed with relocation of patients to a safe area). Staff, patients, and, whenever appropriate, patient families must be kept apprised of the choices contemplated and selected.

The decision to evacuate is not an easy one. By necessity, health care facility evacuations force the adoption of a change in the delivery of health care services along the continuum of care from conventional to contingency to crisis response. The implications of such incidents are not simply focused on the facilities that have to evacuate, but also greatly impact those facilities that receive patient evacuees. It also has a big impact on the surrounding community, as patients often look to hospitals as safe havens and continue to seek medical treatment and care. Moreover, the decision to evacuate a health care facility will always be made with less than the full array of information desired by decision makers. Although never prominently discussed, fiduciary concerns related to the decision to "close the doors" can also figure prominently in the process.

As has been often noted of military decision making under stress, leaders must be careful not to end up fighting the "last war" by using strategies and tools with which they are familiar, but are inappropriate for the current situation. In the case of Hurricane Sandy, the mandatory evacuations ordered the year before for a storm surge that never arrived with Hurricane Irene may have been enough to impart a sense of confidence among health care organization leadership and the belief that all would be fine—a mistake that could have been much more costly. Deciding whether "to stay or go" is not an easy decision to make.

REFERENCES

AAP (American Academy of Pediatrics), ACEP (American College of Emergency Physicians), and ENA (Emergency Nurses Association). 2009. Joint policy statement—guidelines for care of children in the emergency department. *Pediatrics* 124(4):1233-1243. http://aappolicy.aappublications.org/cgi/reprint/pediatrics;124/4/1233.pdf (accessed April 3, 2013).

AHRQ (Agency for Healthcare Research and Quality). 2005. *Altered standards of care in mass casualty events: Bioterrorism and other public health emergencies.* Rockville, MD: AHRQ. http://archive.ahrq.gov/research/altstand/altstand.pdf (accessed March 11, 2013).

Alberts, D. S. 2007. Agility, focus, and convergence: The future of command and control. *The International C2 Journal* 1(1):1-30.

ASPR (Assistant Secretary for Preparedness and Response). 2012a. *Healthcare preparedness capabilities: National guidance for healthcare system preparedness.* Washington, DC: Department of Health and Human Services. http://www.phe.gov/preparedness/planning/hpp/pages/default.aspx (accessed March 29, 2013).

ASPR. 2012b. *National Disaster Medical System.* Washington, DC: Department of Health and Human Services. http://www.phe.gov/preparedness/responders/ndms/Pages/default.aspx (accessed April 3, 2013).

ASPR. 2012c. *Hurricane Sandy—Public health situation updates.* Washington, DC: Department of Health and Human Services. http://www.phe.gov/newsroom/Pages/situpdates.aspx (accessed March 11, 2013).

ASPR. 2013a. *Public health emergency medical countermeasures enterprise.* Washington, DC: Department of Health and Human Services. https://www.phe.gov/Preparedness/mcm/phemce/Pages/default.aspx (accessed March 11, 2013).

ASPR. 2013b. *Hospital Preparedness Program (HPP) measure manual: Implementation guidance for the HPP program measures.* Washington, DC: Department of Health and Human Services. http://www.phe.gov/Preparedness/planning/evaluation/Documents/hpp-bp2-measuresguide-2013.pdf (accessed June 17, 2013).

Barbera, J. A., and A. G. MacIntyre. 2007. *Medical surge capacity and capability: A management system for integrating medical and health resources during large-scale emergencies,* 2nd ed. Washington, DC: Department of Health and Human Services. http://www.phe.gov/preparedness/planning/mscc/handbook/documents/mscc080626.pdf (accessed April 3, 2013).

Barbera, J. A., and A. G. MacIntyre. 2009. *Medical surge capacity and capability: The healthcare coalition in emergency response and recovery.* Washington, DC: Department of Health and Human Services. http://www.phe.gov/preparedness/planning/mscc/documents/mscctier2jan2010.pdf (accessed May 14, 2013).

Bell, D. E. 1982. Regret in decision making under uncertainty. *Operations Research* 30(5):961-981.

Brecher, M. 1979. State behavior in international crisis. *Journal of Conflict Resolution* 23(3):446-480.

Burkle, F. M., Jr., and R. Hayden. 2001. The concept of assisted management of large-scale disasters by horizontal organizations. *Prehospital Disaster Medicine* 16(3):87-96.

Carcamo, C. 2012. Storm forces evacuation of hundreds of New York hospital patients. *Los Angeles Times,* October 30. http://articles.latimes.com/2012/oct/30/nation/la-na-nn-hurricane-sandy-hospital-evacuations-20121030 (accessed April 16, 2013).

CDC (Centers for Disease Control and Prevention). 2011. *Public health preparedness capabilities: National standards for state and local planning.* Atlanta, GA: CDC. http://www.cdc.gov/phpr/capabilities (accessed March 29, 2013).

Cibulsky, S. M., and M. A. Kirk. 2010. *Summary: Symposium on chemical decontamination of humans, final report.* Washington, DC: Department of Homeland Security. http://www.phe.gov/Preparedness/mcm/Documents/summary-chemdecon-20June12.pdf (accessed March 11, 2013).

Degani, A., and E. L. Wiener. 1993. Cockpit checklists: Concepts, design, and use. *Human Factors* 35(2):28-43.

Devereaux, A. V., J. R. Dichter, M. D. Christian, N. N. Dubler, C. E. Sandrock, J. L. Hick, T. Powell, J. A. Geiling, D. E. Amundson, T. E. Baudendistel, D. A. Braner, M. A. Klein, K. A. Berkowitz, J. R. Curtis, and L. Rubinson. 2008. Definitive care for the critically ill during a disaster: A framework for allocation of scarce resources in mass critical care. From a Task Force for Mass Critical Care summit meeting, January 26-27, 2007, Chicago, IL. *Chest* 133(Suppl 5):S51-S66.

DHS (Department of Homeland Security). 2011. *Homeland Security Advisory Council: Community Resilience Taskforce recommendations.* Washington, DC: DHS. http://www.dhs.gov/xlibrary/assets/hsac-community-resilience-task-force-recommendations-072011.pdf (accessed May 3, 2013).

Downey, E. L., K. Andress, and C. H. Schultz. 2013a. Initial management of hospital evacuations caused by Hurricane Rita: A systematic investigation. *Prehospital and Disaster Medicine* 28(3):257-263.

Downey, E. L., K. Andress, and C. H. Schultz. 2013b. External factors impacting hospital evacuation caused by Hurricane Rita: The role of situational awareness. *Prehospital and Disaster Medicine* 28(3):264-271.

EMSA (California Emergency Medical Services Authority). 2007. *Disaster Medical Services Division—Hospital Incident Command System (HICS).* http://www.emsa.ca.gov/hics (accessed March 11, 2013).

FEMA (Federal Emergency Management Agency). 2008a. *Incident command system training: Review material.* Washington, DC: FEMA. http://training.fema.gov/EMIWeb/IS/ICSResource/assets/reviewMaterials.pdf (accessed March 11, 2013).

FEMA. 2008b. *Emergency support function annexes: Introduction.* Washington, DC: FEMA. http://www.fema.gov/pdf/emergency/nrf/nrf-esf-intro.pdf (accessed April 3, 2013).

FEMA. 2010. *Developing and maintaining emergency operations plans: Comprehensive preparedness guide (CPG) 101, Version 2.0.* Washington, DC: FEMA. http://www.fema.gov/pdf/about/divisions/npd/CPG_101_V2.pdf (accessed May 14, 2013).

FEMA. 2011. *A whole community approach to emergency management principles, themes, and pathways for action.* FDOC 104-008-1. Washington, DC: FEMA. http://www.fema.gov/library/viewRecord.do?id=4941 (accessed March 11, 2013).

FEMA. 2013. *National Incident Management System (NIMS).* Washington, DC: FEMA. http://www.fema.gov/emergency/nims (accessed March 11, 2013).

Femino, M., S. Young, and V. C. Smith. 2013. Hospital-based emergency preparedness: Evacuation of the neonatal intensive care unit—the smallest and most vulnerable population. *Pediatric Emergency Care* 29(1):107-113.

Fink, S. 2012. *In hurricane's wake, decisions not to evacuate hospitals raise questions.* http://www.propublica.org/article/in-hurricanes-wake-decisions-not-to-evacuate-hospitals-raise-questions (accessed April 3, 2013).

Flin, R., P. O'Connor, and K. Mearns. 2002. Crew resource management: Improving team work in high reliability industries. *Team Performance Management* 8(3-4):68-78.

GAO (Government Accountability Office). 2006. *Disaster preparedness: Limitations in federal evacuation assistance for health facilities should be addressed.* GAO-06-826. Washington, DC: GAO. http://www.gao.gov/new.items/d06826.pdf (accessed April 3, 2013).

GAO. 2008. *States are planning for medical surge, but could benefit from shared guidance for allocating scarce medical resources.* GAO-08-668. Washington, DC: GAO. http://www.gao.gov/new.items/d08668.pdf (accessed March 11, 2013).

Hansson, S. O. 1996. Decision making under great uncertainty. *Philosophy of the Social Sciences* 26(3):369-386.

Helmreich, R. L., and A. C. Merritt. 1998. *Culture at work: National, organisational and professional influences.* Aldershot, Hampshire, England: Ashgate.

Helmreich, R. L., A. C. Merritt, and J. A. Wilhelm. 1999. The evolution of crew resource management training in commercial aviation. *International Journal of Aviation Psychology* 9(1):19-32.

HHS (Department of Health and Human Services). 2005. *Pandemic Influenza Plan Supplement 11.* www.hhs.gov/pandemicflu/plan/pdf/S11.pdf (accessed April 8, 2013).

Hick, J. L., J. A. Barbera, and G. D. Kelen. 2009. Refining surge capacity: Conventional, contingency, and crisis capacity. *Disaster Medicine and Public Health Preparedness* 3(Suppl 2):S59-S67.

IOM (Institute of Medicine). 2009. *Guidance for establishing crisis standards of care for use in disaster situations: A letter report.* Washington, DC: The National Academies Press. http://www.nap.edu/catalog.php?record_id=12749 (accessed April 3, 2013).

IOM. 2010. *Crisis standards of care: Summary of a workshop series.* Washington, DC: The National Academies Press. http://www.nap.edu/catalog.php?record_id=12787 (accessed April 3, 2013).

IOM. 2012. *Crisis standards of care: A systems framework for catastrophic disaster response.* Washington, DC: The National Academies Press. http://www.nap.edu/openbook.php?record_id=13351 (accessed April 3, 2013).

Jen, H. C., S. B. Shew, J. B. Atkinson, J. T. Rosenthal, and J. R. Hiatt. 2009. Creation of inpatient capacity during a major hospital relocation: Lessons for disaster planning. *Archives of Surgery* 144(9):859-864.

Joynt, G. M., S. Loo, B. L. Taylor, G. Margalit, M. D. Christian, C. Sandrock, M. Danis, Y. Leoniv, and C. L. Sprung. 2010. Coordination and collaboration with interface units. *Journal of Intensive Care Medicine* 36(Suppl 1):S21-S31.

Kearns, R. D. 2011. *Burn surge capacity in the south: What is the capacity of burn centers within the American Burn Association southern region to absorb significant numbers of burn injured patients during a medical disaster?* Medical University of South Carolina: ProQuest Dissertations and Theses.

Keinan, G. 1987. Decision making under stress: Scanning of alternatives under controllable and uncontrollable threats. *Journal of Personality and Social Psychology* 52(3):639-644.

Klein, K. R., P. E. Pepe, F. M. Burkle, N. E. Nagel, and R. E. Swienton. 2008. Evolving need for alternative triage management in public health emergencies: A Hurricane Katrina case study. *Disaster Medicine and Public Health Medicine* 2(Suppl 1):S40-S44.

Kowalski-Trakofler, K. M., and C. Vaught. 2003. Judgment and decision making under stress: An overview for emergency managers. *International Journal of Emergency Management* 1(3):278-289.

Mauro, R., A. Degani, L. Loukopoulos, and I. Barshi. 2012. The operational context of procedures and checklists in commercial aviation. *Proceedings of the Human Factors and Ergonomics Society Annual Meeting* 56(1):758-762.

Merin, O., N. Ash, G. Levy, M. J. Schwaber, and Y. Kriess. 2010. The Israeli field hospital in Haiti: Ethical dilemmas in early disaster response. *New England Journal of Medicine* 362(11):e38.

NCIPC (National Center for Injury Prevention and Control). 2007. *In a moment's notice: Surge capacity for terrorist bombings.* Atlanta, GA: CDC. http://emergency.cdc.gov/masscasualties/pdf/surgecapacity.pdf (accessed June 5, 2013).

NTSB (National Transportation Safety Board). 2007. Motorcoach fire on Interstate 45 during Hurricane Rita evacuation near Wilmar, Texas, September 23, 2005. Highway Accident Report NTSB/HAR-07/01. Washington, DC: NTSB. http://www.ntsb.gov/doclib/reports/2007/HAR0701.pdf (accessed April 12, 2012).

O'Connor, P., J. Campbell, J. Newon, J. Melton, E. Salas, and K. Wilson. 2008. Crew resource management training effectiveness: A meta-analysis and some critical needs. *International Journal of Aviation Psychology* 18(4):353-368.

Ohio Hospital Association and Ohio Department of Health. 2011. *Ohio medical coordination plan.* Columbus: Ohio Hospital Association and Ohio Department of Health.

ORISE (Oak Ridge Institute for Science and Education). 2013a. *Public health discussion guide for pandemic influenza planning.* http://www.cdc.gov/phpr/healthcare/documents/Discussion_Guide_for_Public_Health.pdf (accessed May 15, 2013).

ORISE. 2013b. *Hospital discussion guide for pandemic influenza planning.* http://www.cdc.gov/phpr/healthcare/documents/Discussion_Guide_for_Hospitals.pdf (accessed May 15, 2013).

ORISE. 2013c. *Emergency management discussion guide for pandemic influenza planning.* http://www.cdc.gov/phpr/healthcare/documents/Discussion_Guide_for_Emergency_Management.pdf (accessed May 15, 2013).

Phillips, S. J., and A. Knebel, eds. 2007. *Mass medical care with scarce resources: A community planning guide.* Rockville, MD: AHRQ. http://archive.ahrq.gov/research/mce/mceguide.pdf (accessed June 10, 2013).

Powell, T., K. C. Christ, and G. S. Birkhead. 2008. Allocation of ventilators in a public health disaster. *Disaster Medicine and Public Health Preparedness* 2(1):20-26.

Renaud, C. 2012. The missing piece of NIMS: Teaching incident commanders how to function in the edge of chaos. *Homeland Security Affairs* Article 8. http://www.hsaj.org/?article=8.1.8 (accessed April 22, 2013).

Rosenthal, U., and P. t'Hart. 1991. Experts and decision makers in crisis situations. *Knowledge: Creation, Diffusion, Utilization* 12(4):350-372.

Salas, E., K. A. Wilson, C. S. Burke, and D. C. Wightman. 2006. Does crew resource management training work? An update, an extension, and some critical needs. *Human Factors* 48(2):392-412.

Sarter, N. B., and B. Schroeder. 2001. Supporting decision making and action selection under time pressure and uncertainty: The case of in-flight icing. *Human Factors* 43(4):573-583.

Schultz, C. H., K. L. Koenig, and R. J. Lewis. 2003. Implications of hospital evacuation after the Northridge, California, earthquake. *New England Journal of Medicine* 348(14):1349-1355.

Sexton, K. H., L. M. Alperin, and J. D. Stobo. 2007. Lessons from Hurricane Rita: The University of Texas Medical Branch Hospital's evacuation. *Academic Medicine* 82(8):792-796.

Staal, M. A. 2004. Stress, cognition, and human performance: A literature review and conceptual framework. Hanover, MD: National Aeronautics and Space Administration. http://human-factors.arc.nasa.gov/flightcognition/Publications/IH_054_Staal.pdf (accessed February 11, 2013).

State of Michigan. 2013. *Michigan Emergency Department Syndromic Surveillance System.* Lansing, MI: Department of Community Health. http://www.michigan.gov/mdch/0,4612,7-132-2945_5104_31274-107091--,00.html (accessed April 12, 2013).

Sternberg, E., G. C. Lee, and D. Huard. 2004. Counting crises: US hospital evacuations, 1971-1999. *Prehospital Disaster Medicine* 19(2):150-157.

Subbarao, I., M. K. Wynia, and F. M. Burkle. 2010. The elephant in the room: Collaboration and competition among relief organizations during high-profile disasters. *Journal of Clinical Ethics* 21(4):328-334.

Timbie, J. W., J. S. Ringel, D. S. Fox, D. A. Waxman, F. Pillemer, C. Carey, M. Moore, V. Karir, T. J. Johnson, N. Iyer, J. Hu, R. Shanman, J. W. Larkin, M. Timmer, A. Motala, T. R. Perry, S. Newberry, and A. L. Kellermann. 2012. *Allocation of scarce resources during mass casualty events*. Rockville, MD: AHRQ. http://www.ncbi.nlm.nih.gov/books/NBK98854/pdf/TOC.pdf (accessed June 6, 2013).

Timbie, J. W., J. S. Ringel, D. S. Fox, F. Pillemer, D. A. Waxman, M. Moore, C. K. Hansen, A. R. Knebel, R. Riccardi, and A. L. Kellermann. 2013. Systematic review of strategies to manage and allocate scarce resources during mass casualty events. *Annals of Emergency Medicine* 61(6):677-689.

Walker, I. A., S. Reshamwalla, and I. H. Wilson. 2012. Surgical safety checklists: Do they improve outcomes? *British Journal of Anesthesia* 109(1):47-54.

Winters, B. D., A. P. Gurses, H. Lehmann, J. B. Sexton, C. J. Rampersad, and P. J. Pronovost. 2009. Clinical review: Checklists—translating evidence into practice. *Critical Care* 13(6):210-219.

WHO (World Health Organization). 2009. *Human factors in patient safety: Review of topics and tools*. Geneva, Switzerland: WHO. http://www.who.int/patientsafety/research/methods_measures/human_factors/human_factors_review.pdf (accessed May 20, 2013).

Zaenger, D., N. Efrat, R. R. Riccio, and K. Sanders. 2010. Shelter-in-place versus evacuation decision making: A systematic approach for healthcare facilities. *Risk, Hazards & Crisis in Public Policy* 1(3):19-33.

Zakay, D. 1993. The impact of time perception processes on decision making under time stress. In *Time pressure and stress in human judgment and decision making*, edited by O. Svenson and J. Maule. New York: Plenum. Pp. 59-72.

Zane, R., P. Biddinger, A. Hassol, T. Rich, J. Gerber, and J. DeAngelis. 2010. *Hospital evacuation decision guide*. Rockville, MD: AHRQ. http://archive.ahrq.gov/prep/hospevacguide (accessed April 3, 2013).

2: Indicators and Triggers

On a spring evening, a paramedic witnesses a tornado touch down in town. Debris is flying. The tornado seems to be a perfect indicator (providing discrete information that is certain, and can be easily acted on) to trigger emergency medical services (EMS) and health care organization disaster plan activation. This may be true in a small community. In a large community, additional information is required before making this decision. How big was the tornado? Where did the tornado touch down? Did it primarily affect an industrial park on a Saturday, or a school on a weekday?

The storm system that generated the massive tornado that struck Joplin, Missouri, in 2011 (which appropriately and immediately triggered contingency and crisis responses in the community) also spawned a tornado that struck a neighborhood in Minneapolis, Minnesota. No EMS agencies or hospitals activated their disaster plans as news footage from the scene and early EMS reports indicated mostly minor injuries, all within the scope of conventional operations. Thus, even seemingly ideal indicators may require some processing to determine if a "trigger" threshold has been reached, and these decisions may be directly tied to the resources available in the community. This is why the agency and stakeholder discussions of indicators and triggers outlined in this paper are critical to help understand how indicators can be used to support operational decision making, and when triggers can be automatically activated (scripted), versus those that may require expert analysis prior to a decision (non-scripted).

This chapter examines important concepts and considerations related to indicators and triggers. The material in this chapter will help provide background to the toolkit discussions. The chapter begins by providing definitions and examples of indicators and triggers. Next, the chapter discusses how to develop useful and appropriate indicators and triggers. Following this, the chapter presents some limitations and issues related to indicators. Finally, the chapter discusses systems-level considerations and provides several examples of existing data systems.

WHAT ARE INDICATORS AND TRIGGERS?

Key points: Indicators are measures or predictors of changes in demand and/or resource availability; triggers are decision points. Indicators and triggers guide transitions along the continuum of care, from conventional to contingency to crisis and in the return to conventional.

Indicators and triggers represent the information and actions taken at specific thresholds that guide incident recognition, response, and recovery. Box 2-1 provides definitions; the concepts behind the definitions are discussed in greater detail below.

Indicator information may be available in many forms. Sample indicators and associated triggers and tactics are listed in Table 2-1. More detailed descriptions are available in the discipline-specific discussion toolkits (Chapters 4-9). When specific indicators cross a threshold that is recognized by the community to require action, this represents a trigger point, with actions determined by community plans. These include plans for activation of a general disaster plan, which often occurs at the threshold between conventional and contingency care, and activation of crisis standards of care (CSC) plans, which would occur at the threshold between contingency and crisis care.

DEVELOPING USEFUL INDICATORS AND TRIGGERS

Key points: It can be challenging to identify useful indicators and triggers from among the large and varied sources of available data. Specific numeric "bright line" thresholds for indicators and triggers are concrete and attractive because they are easily recognized, but for many situations the community/agency actions are not as clear-cut or may require significant data analysis before action. Rather than creating a laundry list of possible indicators and triggers, it may be helpful to consider four steps: (1) identify key response strategies and actions, (2) identify and examine potential indicators, (3) determine trigger points, and (4) determine tactics.

The amount of information available in health care today is enormous and expanding. It is attractive to look at many metrics and consider their use as indicators. However, multiple factors may make data monitoring less useful than it originally appears, and it can be challenging to detect or characterize an evolving event amid usual variability in large and complex sets of data (see the "Indicators Limitations and Issues" section below). Specific numeric "bright line" thresholds for indicators and triggers are concrete and attractive because they are easily recognized, and for certain situations they are relatively easy to develop (e.g., a single case of anthrax). However, for many situations the community/agency actions are not as clear-cut or may require significant data analysis to determine the point at which a reasonable threshold may be established (e.g., multiple cases of diarrheal illness in a community).

The accompanying toolkits provide discipline-specific tables and materials to discuss potential indicators and triggers that guide CSC implementation. This section presents key concepts that will help inform the development of these discipline-, agency-, and organization-specific indicators and triggers. Rather than creating a laundry list of possible indicators and triggers, it may be helpful to consider the following four steps. These steps should be considered at the threshold from conventional to contingency care, from contingency to crisis care, and in the return to conventional care. They should also be considered for both slow-onset and no-notice incidents. Subsequent discussion below expands on these steps.

1. *Identify key response strategies and actions* that the facility or agency would use to respond to an incident. (Examples include disaster declaration, establishment of an emergency operations center [EOC] and multiagency coordination, establishment of alternate care sites, and surge capacity expansion.)

BOX 2-1
Definitions

Indicator: A measurement, event, or other data that is a predictor of change in demand for health care service delivery or availability of resources. This may warrant further monitoring, analysis, information sharing, and/or select implementation of emergency response system actions.

>   **Actionable indicator:** An indicator that *can* be impacted through actions taken within an organization or a component of the emergency response system (e.g., a hospital detecting high patient census).

>   **Predictive indicator:** An indicator that *cannot* be impacted through actions taken within an organization or component of the emergency response system (e.g., a hospital receiving notification that a pandemic virus has been detected).

Certain data: Data that require minimal verification and analysis to initiate a trigger.

Uncertain data: Data that require interpretation to determine appropriate triggers and tactics.

Threshold: "A level, point, or value above which something is true or will take place and below which it is not or will not" (Merriam-Webster Dictionary, 2013). A trigger point may be designed to occur at a threshold recognized by the community or agency to require a specific response. Trigger points and thresholds may be the same in many circumstances, but each threshold does not necessarily have an associated trigger.

Trigger: A decision point based on changes in the availability of resources that requires adaptations to health care services delivery along the care continuum (contingency, crisis, and return toward conventional).

>   **Crisis care trigger:** The point at which the scarcity of resources requires a transition from contingency care to crisis care, implemented within and across the emergency response system. This marks the transition point at which resource allocation strategies focus on the community rather than the individual.

>   **Scripted trigger:** A predefined decision point that can be initiated immediately upon recognizing an associated indicator. Scripted triggers lead to scripted tactics.

>   **Non-scripted trigger:** A decision point that requires analysis and leads to implementation of non-scripted tactics.

Scripted tactic: A tactic that is predetermined (i.e., can be listed on a checklist) and is quickly implemented by frontline personnel with minimal analysis.

Non-scripted tactic: A tactic that varies according to the situation; it is based on analysis, multiple or uncertain indicators, recommendations, and, in certain circumstances, previous experience.

TABLE 2-1

Sample Indicators, Triggers, and Tactics by Discipline

Discipline	Indicator	Trigger	Tactic
Emergency management	National Weather Service (NWS) watches/warnings	NWS forecasts Category 4 hurricane landfall in 96 hours	Issue evacuation/shelter orders, determine likely impact, support hospital evacuations with transportation resources, risk communication to public about event impact
Public health	Epidemiology information	Predicted cases exceed epidemic threshold	Risk communication, consideration of need for medical countermeasures/alternate care site planning, establish situational awareness and coordination with EMS/hospitals/long-term care facilities
Emergency medical services (EMS)	911 call	X casualties	Automatic assignment of X ambulances, supervisor, assignment of incident-specific radio talk group
Inpatient	Emergency department (ED) wait times	ED wait times exceed X hours	Increase staffing, diversion of patients to clinics/urgent care, activate inpatient plans to rapidly accommodate pending admissions
Outpatient	Demand forecasting/epidemiology information	Unable to accommodate number of requests for appointments/service	Expand hours and clinic staffing, prioritize home care service provision, increase phone support
Behavioral health	Crisis hotline call volume	Unable to accommodate call volume	Activate additional mental health hotline resources, "immunization" via risk communication, implement psychological first aid (PFA) techniques and risk assessment screening in affected areas

2. *Identify and examine potential indicators* that inform the decision to initiate these actions. (Indicators may be comprised of a wide range of data sources, including, for example, bed availability, a 911 call, or witnessing a tornado.)

3. *Determine trigger points* for taking these actions. Scripted triggers may be derived from certain indicators. If scripted triggers are inappropriate because the indicators require additional assessment and analysis, it will be important to determine the process for arriving at non-scripted triggers (i.e., who is notified/briefed, who provides the assessment and analysis, and who makes the decision to implement the tactic).

4. *Determine tactics* that could be implemented at these trigger points. Scripted triggers may appropriately lead to scripted tactics and a rapid, predefined response.

Predicting every disaster scenario (and related key response strategies, actions, and tactics) is impossible, but following these steps can help focus on key sources of information that act as indicators, and determine whether or not the information supports decisions taken to implement (trigger) specific tactics. These four steps form the basis of the approach taken in this report and will be expanded on in the toolkit with information and examples for each major component of the emergency response system.

Identify Key Response Strategies and Actions

Key point: In planning, organizations and other entities should first determine the response strategies and actions that will be taken in response to an incident.

Rather than jumping straight into enumeration of indicators and triggers, it is valuable to first identify key response strategies and actions, and then consider what indicators and triggers would be most helpful in deciding to implement these response strategies and actions. Key response strategies and actions are determined by community plans:

- Agency/facility triggers into contingency care generally involve activation of facility or agency disaster plans, which produces additional surge capacity that cannot be achieved in conventional response (Barbisch and Koenig, 2006; Hick et al., 2008; Kaji et al., 2006). They are usually agency-/facility-specific due to variability in facility size and resources.
- System-based triggers for coalition, region, or health care system situational awareness, information sharing, and resource management should be established, for example, when more than one coalition facility declares a disaster, when victims are taken to more than three hospitals, or when staff, space, or supply issues are anticipated. There may be significant concordance between regions and coalitions on these triggers, though geographic differences need to be factored in.
- Crisis care triggers tend to be based on exhaustion of specific operational resources that requires a community, rather than an individual, view be taken in regard to resource allocation strategies. Though the threshold may be crossed at an individual facility, it is critical that a system-based response be initiated whenever this occurs in order to diffuse the resource demands and ensure that as consistent a level of care as possible is provided. Most of these triggers will be consistent between facilities and regions and will revolve around lack of appropriate staff, space, or specific supplies. It is important to appreciate that an institutional/agency goal is to avoid reaching a crisis care trigger whenever possible by proactive incident management (i.e., National Incident Management System [NIMS], Hospital Incident Command System [HICS]), and logistics efforts in the facility and region (EMSA, 2007; FEMA, 2013a).

A community may have many more triggers than those noted here that are incorporated in existing emergency response plans (e.g., criteria for second alarm fire, indications for medical director notification, VIP patient protocols). To avoid confusion, trigger discussions should be clarified within the specific operational context (e.g., "crisis care trigger"). Different communities and facilities will clearly have different thresholds based on their resources, and thus similarity of triggers across communities and facilities cannot be assumed; during an incident it is far more helpful to inquire or share details about the specific needs of the facility rather than simply note that a trigger event has occurred (e.g., a circuit breaker trip does not tell the building supervisor what the problem is, just that there may be a problem). Contextual information is important to help frame the specific issue of concern.

Identify and Examine Potential Indicators

Key points: After an agency or a facility determines what actions or strategies are key to its responsibilities during an incident, it should examine and optimize indicator data sources that inform initiation of these actions. Indicator data may be categorized using two primary distinctions: predictive versus actionable and certain versus uncertain. Predictive indicators cannot be directly impacted by actions taken by the agency/facility; actionable indicators are under the control of the agency/facility. An indicator that is actionable for one agency may be predictive for another. Certain data require less analysis before action; uncertain data require interpretation before action. Understanding these characteristics of indicators helps inform decisions about how best to use them.

Indicators and triggers can lead to decisions to implement response tactics along two primary pathways. These two pathways are illustrated in Figure 2-1. One pathway begins with an actionable indicator based on certain data, which could appropriately lead to a scripted[1] trigger and associated scripted (specific, predetermined) tactics. Examples of this first pathway would be a hospital trauma team activation or a first alarm response to report of a fire in a building. A second pathway begins with a predictive indicator based on uncertain data, which would require additional analysis and assessment to reach a non-scripted trigger decision and employment of non-scripted (variable) tactics. An example of this second pathway would be the pathway leading to the declaration of an influenza pandemic. Regardless of the certainty of the data, each pathway passes through a "filter" process in which information is analyzed, assessed, and validated. This process occurs even in the context of certain data, although the filtering requirements are far less than for uncertain data. The remainder of this section uses the figure as a basis for additional discussion of these concepts.

Indicator data may be categorized using two primary distinctions: *predictive* versus *actionable* and *certain* versus *uncertain.*

Predictive indicators can be monitored, but cannot be directly impacted through actions taken within an organization or component of the emergency response system. Examples include monitoring of weather, epidemiologic data, or other such information. Data monitoring at more than one site generally yields information that is predictive, and data monitoring in aggregate may be of use from a system coordination viewpoint (e.g., epidemiology data that drive treatment decision making, system capacity in a large health care system) rather than at the facility level, where data monitoring is less likely to yield information that is not already evident to the providers.

In contrast, *actionable* indicators are under the control of an agency or a facility (and usually only actionable at that level; the more these data are aggregated, generally the less specific and actionable they become). Examples of these types of data are staffed hospital bed capacity, emergency department (ED) wait times, and other operational data that may be affected directly by actions such as increasing staffed beds or activating call-back of personnel.

An indicator that is actionable for one agency may be predictive for another. For example, prolonged ED wait times at a local hospital are actionable for the hospital itself, but they are predictive for the local public health agency (as the agency cannot directly influence the indicator).

---

[1] In business and engineering, these are often referred to as programmed/non-programmed triggers. The committee believed that because these terms did not have wide usage in the public and medical preparedness communities, they should be tied to the scripted and non-scripted tactics for consistency and ease of understanding. See Box 1-5 in Chapter 1 for additional discussion about decision making in crises.

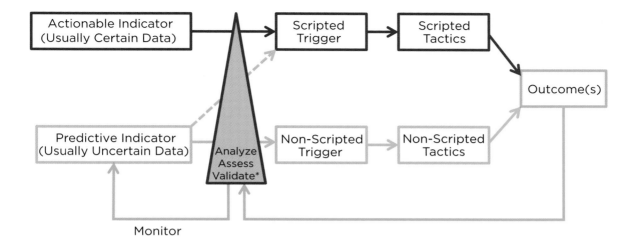

FIGURE 2-1

Relationships among indicators, triggers, and tactics.

*Interpret indicators, other available data, impact, and resources—this may occur over minutes (e.g., developing an initial response to a fire) or days (e.g., developing a response to the detection of a novel virus).

NOTE: In this figure, an indicator is comprised of either certain data, sufficient to activate a trigger, or uncertain data, which require additional analysis prior to action. It is important to note several characteristics that may be helpful in shaping planning:

- All actions require at least minimal validation of data or processing of data—the triangle at the center of the figure shows the relative amount of processing expertise and time required (i.e., the thicker base of the triangle represents more processing required).
- Indicators that are actionable typically involve certain data that can lead to scripted triggers that staff can initiate without further analysis (e.g., if a mass casualty incident involves >20 victims, the mass casualty incident [MCI] plan is activated).
- Indicators that are predictive (e.g., epidemiology data) typically involve uncertain data that require interpretation prior to "trigger" action.
- The smaller the community or the fewer resources available, the more certain and scripted the triggers can become.
- The larger the community (or state/national level) and the more resources available, the less certain the data become as they do not reflect significant variability in resource availability at the local level—thus, the more expert interpretation is often required prior to action (e.g., state level data may reveal available beds, but select facilities and/or jurisdictions may be far beyond conventional capacity).
- The larger or more direct the impact, the more certain the data (e.g., when the tornado hits your hospital, there is no question you should trigger your disaster plan and implement contingency or crisis care tactics as required).
- Scripted triggers are quickly implemented by frontline personnel with minimal analysis—the disadvantage is that the scripted tactics may commit too few or too many resources to the incident (e.g., first alarm response to report of a fire in a building).
- Non-scripted triggers are based on expert analysis rather than a specific threshold and allow implementation of tactics that are tailored to the situation (non-scripted tactics). Trigger decisions may be based on expertise, experience, indicator(s) interpretation, etc., and may be made quickly or take significant time based on the information available.
- Ongoing monitoring and additional analysis of indicators will help assess the current situation and the impact of the tactics.

The data on which indicators are based may be *certain* (requiring less analysis) or *uncertain* (requiring interpretation prior to action). Most predictive indicators tend to be based on uncertain data, though in some cases enough certain data are provided to make immediate decisions (e.g., tornado directly hits a hospital). Actionable indicators usually are based on certain data. It is important to note that decision making in crises often requires acting on uncertain information. The fact that information is uncertain means that additional assessment and analysis may be required, but this should not impede the ability to plan and act.

The utility of the indicator should be considered separately from the utility of the available data; for example, while bed availability may be a useful indicator, the available data in a community may not be useful if they are of poor quality. Indicator and data limitations are discussed further below. When data are required to make decisions, the following issues may help frame higher-level or interagency discussion. The discipline-specific discussions later in the report provide more specific key questions.

- What are the key agency decisions and actions relative to disaster declarations and entering crisis standards of care?

- What is the rationale for the use of data to inform these decisions and actions?
- When are data needed (prior to the incident, during, or both)?
- Are the data currently available? (If not, how easily are they gathered and reported? If so, from what source, and how timely are the data?)
- Will the data be accurate? (E.g., do data rely on active data entry, or are they passively collected from electronic systems such as electronic medical records? Are they being reported the same way from all entities?)
- How will the data be collected/used/shared/processed/analyzed (including consideration of issues of proprietary information, concerns about the ability of state agencies to "take" reported assets, etc.)?
- How do the data drive actions? If the data do not affect agency/facility actions, they likely are not worthwhile collecting unless they are of greater benefit to public health in aggregate (and the facility will receive feedback on the information provided).

Determine Triggers and Tactics

Key points: After an agency or a facility has determined potential indicators, the facility or agency should identify trigger points and actions that should be taken when the trigger is reached. This includes considering the extent to which the indicators need to be analyzed prior to action and determining whether scripted (predetermined) triggers and tactics are appropriate or whether the triggers should be non-scripted and customized to the situation. It is important to strike a balance between enabling quick action when time is of the essence, but not "overscripting" when time will allow the tactics to be more closely tailored to the situation. It is also important to define who is notified about indicators, who analyzes the indicator data, and who can act on that information.

This section discusses the analysis, assessment, and validation of indicators, and outlines considerations for determining whether there are scripted triggers and tactics that can be employed, or whether the triggers and tactics should be non-scripted and incident-specific.

Analyze, Assess, and Validate

All data require some validation or interpretation, however minimal, prior to activating a trigger based on the data. This may be as simple as understanding the reliability of a data feed, making a phone call to confirm, or asking additional questions of a 911 caller. Some data require significant validation. For example, an indicator of gastroenteritis in a community that achieves a threshold may require significant epidemiological investigation just to determine whether the presence of disease in the community is a valid indicator of a sentinel event, or simply represents a coincidence or normal variant.

For no-notice disaster incidents, the initial indicator is often a 911 call reporting a mass casualty incident, and all that remains is determining a threshold for the dispatcher to trigger the mass casualty plan for the agency. For slow-onset (e.g., pandemic, flood, hurricane) incidents it may not be as simple, and multiple factors may have to be considered when weighing decisions about clinical care, hospital evacuation, etc.

Defining who analyzes and can act on the uncertain data (and how the indicator comes to their attention) is very important. These personnel should have sufficient expertise to consider resources available, time of day, etc., in making their decision—for example, a hospital physician with authority to activate the facility disaster plan hears that a tornado has touched down somewhere in the community. In a large community with multiple hospitals, no disaster plan activation may be needed on a Tuesday at 3 p.m., for example, but if media reports show major damage and it is Saturday evening, the trigger for the hospital disaster plan should be pulled.

Scripted and Non-Scripted Triggers

Indicators that provide rationale for informed decision making may lead to the ability to set thresholds for analysis or trigger actions. The following questions are useful to consider for each indicator that is considered relevant to agency/facility actions:

- Is there a relevant trigger threshold for this resource/category?
- Is it based on an incident report, or based on resource use/capacity?
- Is it predictable enough to act as a trigger?
- How often will the trigger threshold be reached? (If the trigger threshold is rarely reached, a certain degree of oversensitivity/overresponse is appropriate.)
- What actions are required when the trigger is reached (activation of disaster plan, opening of EOC, triage of resources)?
- Are these actions congruent with other agencies/facilities in the area? (Triggers will not be identical due to differences in facility/agency resources, but the actions taken should be congruent—see further discussion below.)

It is important to strike a balance with triggers of taking appropriate action, but not to "overscript" triggers when time is not of the essence. An example of this can be seen in the decision taken by the World Health Organization during the 2009 H1N1 pandemic. They chose not to declare H1N1 a pandemic for some time, even though it met all of the established criteria. They withheld the declaration because of the limited severity of the disease (Garrett, 2009; WHO, 2011). This can create confusion and inconsistencies, and thus a range of response options should be specified when the actions taken require a level of analysis, and the impact and data are less certain.

Triggers may be scripted or non-scripted; Table 2-2 presents a comparison of the properties of each type of trigger. Scripted triggers are very helpful when time is of the essence. They are usually based on information that is certain enough for frontline personnel to take action without significant analysis. For example, checklists and standard operating procedures may specify scripted "if/then" actions and tactics such as

- Fire on a hospital unit = evacuate patients to adjacent smoke-free compartment
- Mass casualty incident (MCI) involving more than 10 victims = activate EMS MCI plan
- Health alert involving novel illness = notify emergency management group

The disadvantage of scripted triggers is that they sometimes will not match the resources to the incident well. Scripted triggers should be designed in a conservative fashion so that they are more likely to overcommit, rather than undercommit, resources relative to the scope of the incident. This is acceptable when

TABLE 2-2
Properties of Scripted and Non-Scripted Triggers

	Scripted	Non-Scripted
Indicator	Actionable (or select predictive indicators, usually in extreme incidents)	Predictive (rarely actionable, especially when multiple data streams or unclear impact)
Data	Certain	Uncertain
Analysis	Minimal	Significant
Simplicity	Yes	No
Speed	Yes	No[a]
Tactics	Scripted	Non-scripted
Demand/resource matching	No	Yes

[a] Though processing time may be brief, depending on the situation.

the activation is rare, and if delay has a high potential to have a negative impact on life safety. The more often the trigger is used, the more refinement is required so the scripted tactics better match resources to the historical incident demands. It is important to note that the trigger action may simply be that a line employee provides scripted emergency notifications to a team or an individual that will then determine further actions (rather than the trigger activating the actual response actions). Box 2-2 provides an example of how a medium-sized health care coalition region might approach determining a dispatch-based scripted trigger threshold for activation of disaster plans.

Non-scripted triggers are more appropriate when at least one of the following is present:

- There is time to make an analytical decision (e.g., usually *not* no-notice, or at least some processing of information required);
- Multiple indicators are involved;
- Demand/resource analysis is required;
- Tiered response is possible which can tailor the resources to achieve the desired outcome(s) (demand/resource matching) and does not introduce unacceptable delay; and/or
- Expertise is required to interpret the potential impact of the indicator.

Scripted and Non-Scripted Tactics

Facility-level crisis care triggers should activate resources and plans rather than specific actions (e.g., not automatically implement triage of resources). For example, though no available ventilators may be a crisis care trigger, it does not mean that ventilator triage should immediately commence. The trigger action should reflect that incident command should immediately work with subject matter experts, logistics, and supporting agencies to determine

- Time frame for obtaining additional resources;
- Potential to transfer patients to facilities with ventilators;
- Utility of bag-valve ventilation or other potential strategies; and
- Process for triage of resources if appropriate.

BOX 2-2
EMS Example Dispatch-Based Scripted Trigger Threshold

This table provides an example of how a medium-sized region might approach determining a dispatch-based scripted trigger threshold for activation of disaster plans. It is not all-inclusive and does not reflect specifics of all jurisdictions. School bus, wheelchair, and other vehicles may need to be included. HAZMAT and other complicating factors may change assumptions. Regulatory and other processes may need to be addressed when activating a mass casualty incident (MCI) plan. These calculations are provided as an example only.

	Agency	Region
Emergency medical services (EMS) units staffed	15	200
EMS units unstaffed	2	15
Mass casualty incident (MCI) buses	0	2 (20 patients per bus)
Private basic life support (BLS) units	0	12

Assumptions:
- Day and night staffing and delay time to staff unstaffed units may have to be factored in
- Unit hour utilization data show 1/3 of units on average are available at a given time = 5 units agency, approximately 60 units regionally
- Other agency units should be able to clear within 45 minutes = 10
- Each ambulance can transport two patients in a disaster
- Round-trip time = 45 minutes per unit

Agency capacity of 44 patients in first 90 minutes—but initial capacity of 10—second wave of transports depends on mutual aid to respond or backfill usual calls.

Regional capacity approximately 120 patients in first 60 minutes (assumes longer response time for mutual aid units). With activation of disaster plan + 40 for MCI buses + 24 for privates = 164 patients/45 minutes after first 45 minutes (assume activation time for MCI buses and private units, and MCI bus turnaround time 90 minutes due to longer loading/unloading time).

Thus consider >10 significantly injured victims as trigger for agency disaster plan and >125 patients trigger for regional plan (would exceed ability to address with simple mutual aid response).

De Boer defines a "Medical Assistance Chain" from medical rescue to medical transport and hospital care where for EMS capacity is estimated by N × S / C. N is number of injured, S is severity (nonambulatory), and C is transport capacity. This construct may be helpful to frame discussion around transport methods and resources (de Boer) and has been refined by Bayram and colleagues—both of these theoretical frameworks include potentially valuable considerations for hospitals as well (Bayram and Zuabi, 2012; Bayram et al., 2012; de Boer, 1999).

In a longer-duration incident, conditions of contingency and crisis are likely to fluctuate across multiple variables, specifically time, disciplines, and resources. For example, EMS agencies during nighttime hours may be operating under contingency or even conventional response conditions, but during daytime peak hours they are consistently applying crisis care tactics. Another example in hospitals or the outpatient setting may be encountered when an organization faces initial limitations of basic supplies, followed by later restrictions in staff availability. The importance of specific triggers under these dynamic conditions becomes less relevant, as the resources available are used to their maximum benefit in the context of an ongoing incident management process. New and incident-specific triggers may be created during this process if required (e.g., if flood crest forecast exceeds 20 feet, commence facility evacuation) and are always best if advance planning can be implemented based on a Hazard Vulnerability Analysis.

Education and Training

Key point: Implementation of actions depends on the level of training and authority and requires appropriate education.

All of the following groups must be integrated into CSC planning and response:

- Frontline employees: Awareness—actions should be scripted at specific thresholds and be made as concrete as possible (e.g., activate EMS disaster plan for MCI involving >10 victims). Awareness may also be an appropriate goal for elected officials and executive officers.
- Supervisors: Knowledge—initial triggers and tactics should be scripted, but with some flexible interpretation of the trigger threshold (disaster declaration for hospital by nursing supervisor or ED physician) and perhaps simple, phased-response options.
- Managers/directors: Proficiency—trigger should be scripted for notification and activation of incident management process, but tactics can be non-scripted and based on expert analysis of the situation with subject matter expert input. This often requires regional/coalition consistency and coordination (e.g., decisions about how to manage limited availability of N95 masks).

Return to Conventional Care

Key point: As conditions improve, it is important to plan and watch for indicators that the system can move back toward conventional care status.

Indicators of return to conventional care may be incident-specific and not included in an agency's usual data or list of indicators. Examples of these indicators are listed in the discipline-specific tables in the toolkit section and may include

- Decreasing call volumes or demands for services;
- Restored systems (utilities, etc.); and
- Decreasing use of hotlines, dispensing sites, alternate care centers, etc.

These variables may fluctuate over the course of a disaster response, as noted in the EMS example above—so return to conventional may be temporary or episodic. Return to conventional care status is not the same as recovery, although it may be an indicator of transition into the recovery phase. Recovery implies a more permanent return to normal operating status and the restoration of the impacted systems and communities. Thus, demobilization of resources should not be dependent on scripted triggers because a return to conventional operations or a decrease in volume of hotline calls or other markers may be temporary, and may be affected by high-profile illness deaths, or other factors.

A more difficult decision-making process occurs when the resources that are supplied to the disaster area provide more resources than were present prior to the incident (e.g., critical care services after the Haiti earthquake, or unified health, medical, mental health, and social work support at shelters for disaster victims). The decisions to withdraw these resources can be difficult, and especially in these cases, thresholds for demobilization should be considered early in the incident; every effort should be made to provide services that can be sustained after the departure of the assets (Kirsch et al., 2012; Subbarao et al., 2010).

INDICATOR LIMITATIONS AND ISSUES

As the discussion above makes clear, the use of indicators and data is not always straightforward. This section briefly presents a number of limitations and issues associated with indicators that stakeholders should keep in mind when developing plans for indicators and associated triggers.

Accuracy

Key point: Indicators are only as valid as the accuracy of the data being considered.

If the data are bad (outdated, not accurate—due to not having the same understanding of what to report or poor data entered—or simply not reported), then they cannot inform good decisions. As noted above, validating data before acting is important, even if this step is done very quickly.

Reporting Data in a Dynamic and Complex Environment

Key points: When developing and using indicators, it is important to be aware of the "rules of reporting," of naming conventions, and that the data are being reported in a dynamic and complex environment.

The "rules of reporting" used and the naming conventions applied during an incident may affect the value of indicators. For example, only a few intensive care beds may be available in a given city, but by activation of surge plans, many more beds may be made available just by staffing currently unstaffed beds or using postanesthesia care units (Devereaux et al., 2008; Rivara et al., 2006; Sprung et al., 2010). Or zero ventilators may be listed as available, but this may not consider the availability and use of transport ventilators, anesthesia machines, or other resources. So, even certain numbers based on actionable data do not necessarily yield scripted triggers for crisis care (though for both of these examples, reaching such a threshold should still prompt action to assess and address the situation, as these are still relevant predictive indicators of system capacity problems, and proactive management decisions are strongly preferred to reactive ones made when there is no option left but crisis care). Who is alerted in these situations, performs this analysis, and decides whether to initiate a trigger based on the information is a key component of agency/facility plans. When indicators are compared or aggregated, the definitions must be the same: If, under "beds available," one jurisdiction counts unstaffed beds and another does not, or if critical access hospitals list monitored beds in the "ICU" category, the dataset is far less useful.

Similarly, it is important to be aware of the dynamic environment in which data reporting is occurring. Even in data-sharing systems that are considered to provide "real-time" data to support situational awareness and crisis decision making (examples are discussed below), there is an important caveat. In each of these systems, there is a time lag between acquiring primary data points, verification of the data received, and reporting that information. Many emergency operations centers and health care coalitions are maturing to the point of developing an information clearinghouse function that can serve to collect and collate such information, but the reporting must be recognized as representing static data points in what is very often a very dynamic environment. This can be illustrated using the same "bed reporting" example used above. The description of actual bed numbers in a preincident collection of data usually reflects either licensed or "staffed" beds (conventional surge response), but not what might be available under contingency or crisis response (DeLia, 2006). For example, intensive care units (ICUs) that run at or near capacity most of the time will only ever report a few beds under conventional (preincident) conditions. But if an incident, sudden or not, were to occur, additional ICU beds located in shuttered units, surgical recovery, or "step-down" units would all be quickly available (assuming staff would also be rapidly mobilized to support the care of patients in these areas), and selected patients would be moved out of ICU beds to intermediate care areas. The information that the local and state authorities choose to gather should be best oriented toward functional reporting, rather than resource reporting, whenever possible. For example, functional capability regarding health care facility response may include reports not just of "beds," but the resources that accompany the placement of patients in those beds—specialized staff, necessary equipment, supplies, and pharmaceuticals.

Separating Signal from Noise

Key point: In considering a data source as an indicator, it is important to consider whether it is feasible to extract actionable information or detect an evolving event from the data source.

For some indicators, separating *signal* from *noise* (i.e., detecting actionable information or characterizing an evolving event amid standard variability in large and complex sets of data) can be challenging, particularly for incidents that develop slowly, such as a pandemic influenza. Boxes 2-3 and 2-4 discuss the promise and perils of using technology, modeling, and social media to predict and detect a surge in demand in real-time. Box 2-3 discusses modeling to predict and detect surge in hospitals, and Box 2-4 discusses these issues as related to influenza pandemic.

Time Required for Reporting

Key point: Automating information exchange and focusing on key information that drives actions will help reduce the demand on staff time during a response.

Requests for resource information is often a distraction from response efforts, or may end up serving as an unintentional drain of limited staff-hours available to attend to specific requests. The less value the facility or agency sees in reporting the data, the less likely the data will be timely or accurate. Automating information exchange, where key data can be pulled or pushed without having to use significant human resources to prepare such data, would help avoid this concern. This issue would be addressed in information-sharing systems by ensuring the interoperability of the data captured by these systems, and by minimizing differences in vendors and proprietary systems that interfere with the exchange of key information.

SYSTEMS-LEVEL CONSIDERATIONS FOR INDICATORS AND TRIGGERS

Key point: Integrated planning among all major components of the emergency response system is critical for an effective and coordinated response.

This section outlines system-level considerations for indicators and triggers; Chapter 1 provides additional discussion of the systems approach to catastrophic disaster response.

Use of Indicators and Data at Different Levels of the Emergency Response System

Key points: Data that may be very actionable at the agency or facility level may be only of limited use in regional aggregate. Data that are valuable at one tier of the medical response may not have immediate value at another level.

Bed occupancy and other data that may be very actionable at the agency or facility level may be of only limited use in regional aggregate, especially when facilities are disproportionately affected (e.g., children's hospitals) and these stresses are not reflected in overall system data or shared among the health care coalitions statewide. However, all data do not have to be used for indicators and triggers in order to be valuable. The data may still have significant value, particularly for overall system capacity monitoring during an incident. Those responsible for regional- or state-level assessment and monitoring should understand that most of the data available to them will be predictive, and that their indicators and triggers may be different from those for the local community. Regional entities, particularly those elements that serve as the command and control function for health care coalitions, such as the Regional Medical Coordination Center, must also assume the role of ensuring the timeliness and validity of data provided (Burkle et al., 2007). In this manner, the coalition serves the important function of providing a clearinghouse for vetting and exchanging useful information.

Data that are valuable at one tier of the medical response may not have immediate value at another level. For example, during the 2009 H1N1 pandemic, King County, Washington, collected a 30-item dataset on intensive care patients with influenza (King County et al., 2009). These data for the most part would not aid the facility response and would be of limited utility at the community level. However, had the same data been collected in real time statewide or nationwide and analyzed by subject matter experts, it might have provided critical treatment information for future cases that could have been shared nationally to influence the overall response. This is why stakeholder collaborative discussion is critical to understanding what data are useful at what level, and requires commitment to supplying the data according to the documented needs and use.

Agencies and facilities supplying data should have a clear understanding of who can access their data, how the data are used, and how the agencies and facilities will benefit by providing the data. In some cases,

BOX 2-3
Promise and Limitations 1: Hospital Surge Capacity

Extensive work has been done on recognizing and forecasting emergency department (ED) daily surge and crowding (Schweigler et al., 2009; Wiler et al., 2011). Although the emergency and trauma care system is often stretched and temporary surges may exacerbate issues such as chronic ED crowding, boarding, and ambulance diversion, and may stress resources and staff, hospitals generally maintain usual standards of care during these times (IOM, 2007a,b). It is recognized that the use of the term *surge capacity* in mass casualty incidents is not equated with daily variations in ED volume, although there may be some relationship (Davidson et al., 2006; Handler et al., 2006; Jenkins et al., 2006). One key problem has been extrapolating factors to daily fluctuations in patient surge—for which there are good data—to disaster situations, where the data are sparse.

Unfortunately, although there is some increasingly useful information about how ED throughput is affected by other factors such as inpatient capacity and rate of presentation, it is clear that many interdependent variables exist, and that daily management of surge is not disaster (and certainly not catastrophic disaster) modeling (Jenkins et al., 2006; McCarthy et al., 2008).

Handler and colleagues (2006) proposed 13 potential data points for studying surge capacity, though this was expert opinion–based and these data points have not been tested for validity. They recognized the deficit of data that are available and can be shared, concluding that they recognize

> the need to make data available to clinicians, administrators, public health officials, and internal and external systems; the importance of real-time data, data standards, and electronic transmission; seamless integration of data capture into the care process; the value of having data available from a single point of access through which data mining, forecasting, and modeling can be performed; and the basic necessity of a criterion standard metric for quantifying surge capacity. (Handler et al., 2006, p. 1173)

Seven years after these conclusions were published, no progress has been made toward these goals.

Furthermore, there are really three types of surge that require different assumptions and responses (Jenkins et al., 2006):

1. Large numbers of patients presenting over a brief period;
2. Sustained increases in volume; and
3. Small numbers of patients with extensive demands for complex, resource-intensive specialty services.

Most of the modeling that is helpful operationally for hospitals revolves around the first of these types of surge. The rate of ED arrivals has been discussed as a key metric (Bayram et al., 2011; Bradt et al., 2009; Hirschberg et al., 2005) and daily marker (McCarthy et al., 2006) of surge, though it is clear that inpatient capacity has a significant effect as well, causing efficiency to decrease as census increases (Asplin et al., 2006).

There seems to be some modeling concordance around 15 seriously injured patients/hour (or ED beds/3.75) as being severely stressful on a trauma center (Bayram et al., 2011; Hirschberg et al., 2005), which aligns with work by de Boer (1999) that estimated 2-3 patients/100 hospital beds/hour could be accommodated with hospital disaster plan activation. Notably, this rate carried over 6 hours approximates 20 percent of hospital bed capacity for most centers, which is consistent with Israeli planning targets (Israel Ministry of Health, 1976; Kosashvili et al., 2009; Tadmor et al., 2006) and accommodates the vast majority of mass casualty incidents. See Peleg and Kellermann (2009) for additional information on Israel's system for hospital surge capacity and for notifying hospitals about the approximate number and type of casualties to anticipate.

Some relevant time-phase work has been done with data from bombings and other no-notice mass casualty incidents, where 50 percent of the victims presented to hospitals within the first hour and the vast majority within 3 hours (CDC, 2003, 2010). This may be helpful as the hospital command center opens to provide some assumptions about what degree of resources may be required over what span of time.

Significant variation for calculating inpatient numbers and capacity also has been noted, depending on how beds are counted, reinforcing that data may be falsely alarming or reassuring (DeLia, 2006; Schull, 2006). Determining the impact that longer-term incidents may have is also very difficult because the modeling for pandemic influenza ranges from minimal to catastrophic impacts on the health care system. Nevertheless, some evidence shows that efficient use of beds within a regional system may save lives in a major disaster (Kanter, 2007) and that these types of coordinated efforts at the coalition and state levels are worthwhile and can make a difference.

Data on "surge discharge" is improving, with several articles reflecting the ability to discharge 30 to 60 percent of patients (Challen and Walter, 2006; Kelen et al., 2006, 2009; Satterthwaite and Atkinson, 2012). These percentages may vary depending on the patient population and size of the facility, but surge discharge clearly represents a critical part of hospital surge response. Hospital planners should have a good idea about baseline capacity that can be generated for their facility and have a plan to rapidly implement these techniques. Improved electronic health records systems may allow anticipated discharges or potential discharge status to be reflected on a daily basis, greatly facilitating decision making in a disaster.

As hospitals gain experience with incidents such as the 2009 H1N1 pandemic, they can determine how those historic volumes were managed and apply these metrics and strategies to future incidents. As electronic records systems grow more robust, passive data analysis and submission to central databases may allow the development of much better predictive modeling that can account for disaster demands as well as daily demands. Regional and state agency stakeholders should look for opportunities to partner with hospitals in these areas of meaningful use of encounter and clinical data.

BOX 2-4
Promise and Limitations 2: Pandemic Influenza

Traditional influenza surveillance programs are conducted by the Centers for Disease Control and Prevention (CDC) primarily to gain an understanding of the nature of the influenza viruses, extent of disease activity, current impact on hospitalizations, and mortality (CDC, 2012b). *FluView*, a weekly influenza surveillance report that provides data on national and regional levels with a lag of 1-2 weeks, is produced from these data (CDC, 2013).

In recent years additional data streams and modeling have been used to supplement traditional surveillance, including pharmacy sales, calls to emergency services, work or school attendance, insurance and billing claims, search data, social media, telephone medical hotlines, and websites specifically aimed at providing information regarding the severity of symptoms and recommended care to seek (e.g., Espino et al., 2003; IOM, 2012b; Kellermann et al., 2010; Koonin and Hanfling, 2013; Magruder et al., 2004; Price et al., 2013; Rolland et al., 2006). This box discusses some of the issues related to mining non-traditional sources of information to guide decision making along the continuum of care (for more extensive reviews of syndromic surveillance system usage, benefits, and limitations, see, for example, Buehler and colleagues [2008, 2009] and IOM and NRC [2011]). Novel approaches offer the potential to provide earlier detection, demand, and severity forecasting, and faster surge detection. Much of this work has been done on influenza, but could be applied to other slow-onset situations, though [it] would not likely be as helpful for no-notice incidents.

Geographic information system–based mapping tools (Google Earth) combined with other data inputs, including social media crowd-source reporting, are also being used to enhance the ability of response agencies to build a picture of what is occurring closer to real time (e.g., Brownstein et al., 2009, Schmidt, 2012). Projects such as HealthMap (2013), founded by a team of researchers, epidemiologists, and software developers at Boston Children's Hospital in 2006, serve as an example of using available online sources to monitor disease outbreaks and provide real-time surveillance of emerging public health threats. MedMap (ASPR, 2013) is another tool, available to local, state, and federal public health and emergency health care response agencies. It is intended to develop a common operating platform for shared health care system resource information, which can be layered onto other response and demographic information data. This can be used to improve situational awareness and the decision making that follows from the availability of such information. It allows for the visualization of special data, with inputs and data point assessments determined by the user of the system, tailoring information inputs to those that are most likely to help inform decision making during large-scale incidents.

The most prominent Web data mining effort is Google Flu Trends (GFT) (2013). Other examples include monitoring and soliciting Twitter users to track disease activity (MappyHealth, 2013; Sickweather, 2013; Signorini et al., 2011) and active data entry programs for individuals such as *Flu Near You* (2013).

GFT, which is the most studied of the Web data mining efforts, illustrates some of the promise and peril with these novel data sources. GFT estimates prevalence from search engine queries for flu-related terms (GFT, 2013). In many cases, GFT estimates have closely matched estimates derived from the traditional surveillance efforts led by CDC, and can be delivered 7-10 days faster (Carneiro and Mylonakis, 2009; Ginsberg et al., 2009; Polgreen et al., 2008). However, in the 2012-2013 influenza season, GFT's estimate of the peak was nearly double the CDC's estimate based on traditional surveillance data (Butler, 2013). GFT also underestimated influenza-like illness (ILI) at the start of the 2009 Influenza A (H1N1) pandemic, requiring an algorithm tweak (Cook et al.,

2011). Other work has suggested that while GFT may correlate well with ILI rates, it may not correlate with actual influenza virus infections (Ortiz et al., 2011). GFT algorithms will undoubtedly continue to evolve (Butler, 2013).

Dugas and colleagues (2013) developed an influenza forecast model based on easy-to-access data that are available in real time, including at individual medical centers. They also incorporated GFT meteorological and temporal information. The best model was able to predict weekly influenza cases within seven cases for 83 percent of estimates for a large urban tertiary center emergency department (ED) in Baltimore. This model may help guide prediction of surge response, but additional evaluation is needed on generalizability. It also remains vulnerable to mismatches between the GFT and traditional surveillance data.

To date, GFT has been used primarily to spur increased vigilance, further investigation, and collection of direct measures, and not as a basis for operational actions (Carneiro and Mylonakis, 2009; Ginsberg et al., 2009). City-level GFT data have been shown to correlate with both positive influenza test results and the volume of ED visits with ILI (Dugas et al., 2012), and may offer some promise in forecasting. The GFT data also correlated well with certain ED crowding measures for pediatric patients and moderately for low-acuity adult patients, but not for higher acuity adult patients. GFT is susceptible to false alerts caused by increased queries due to media attention, for example, but because GFT correlated with ED visits, it may still be useful for surge planning even if the increase is due to enhanced concern rather than an actual increase in influenza prevalence (Dugas et al., 2012).

Temporal relation between ED visits and contact with telehealth lines are other examples of indicators. In Ontario, Canada, call volume to Telehealth Ontario showed that increases in call volume correlated with increases in discharge diagnosis data for respiratory illnesses (van Dijk et al., 2008). Telehealth Ontario data are available electronically in near real time. Additional modeling work found that Telehealth Ontario call volume data can be used to estimate future ED visits for respiratory illness at the health unit level, of which there are 36 in Ontario (Perry et al., 2010). Forecast accuracy was better for health units with a population of more than 400,000. An important limitation is that if the hotline is promoted or referenced in the media, the model predictions may not be accurate because they are tied to prior ED visits.

Other efforts have been made to develop statistical models that predict the severity of the influenza season based on sequence and serological data (Wolf et al., 2010). This study found that these types of data could be used to predict severity. Because the scale of this model is North America, geographically, and based on an entire season, temporally, this type of model may have promise for informing vaccine selection and manufacturing; however, at this point it is unlikely to be useful for operational planning at the health system, organization, or agency level.

The methods and models discussed above show the potential promise of novel techniques and modeling for earlier detection, severity prediction, and demand forecasting. These underlying algorithms and models will undoubtedly continue to improve. However, at this point these are probably not a source of information that could be used as indicators and triggers to drive operational planning and decision making. Furthermore, the application is limited to slow-onset diseases with high prevalence across large populations. Currently most work is focused just on influenza, and outputs are subject to significant error. A final gap is that the United States has no system to share standard clinical information sets and no way to have clinicians collaborate electronically to gather rapidly evolving best practices in real time. Hopefully this can be addressed through official and unofficial channels in advance of the next pandemic or severe seasonal influenza year.

it may be necessary to aggregate data in reporting to avoid singling out organizations or entities, or necessary to specify which offices at a health department have access to the data.

Utility by Jurisdiction Size

Key point: The utility of specific indicators will vary significantly by jurisdiction.

In many urban areas, even large numbers of simultaneous casualties (e.g., the 2013 bombing in Boston, Massachusetts) or catastrophic community damage (e.g., the 2013 Moore, Oklahoma, tornado) do not require implementation of crisis standards of care because of the resiliency within the area emergency response systems. Because of the scale of resources available in urban versus rural settings, many indicators may be of limited utility in rural areas. For example, bed counts at critical access hospitals are not likely to yield much useful information if that is the only reasonable destination for EMS transport units. A recent survey found that 95 percent of rural facilities would be overwhelmed by 10 patients with serious injuries, which was consistent with the EMS estimated response capability (Furbee et al., 2006; Manley et al., 2006). However, due to this paucity of resources, it may be even more critical to be able to develop scripted triggers and tactics that can enable assistance to be mobilized without delay by line personnel (dispatchers, first responders, etc.) and thus support response with available resources and early mobilization of mutual aid.

Goals at Different Levels of the Emergency Response System

Key point: Different types of indicators may be most valuable at different levels of the system.

Because of the dynamic and complex environment in which information is being collected and shared, as described above, it is valuable to focus on a few key system indicators, rather than trying to monitor "everything at once." This section outlines the types of indicators that may be most valuable at different levels of the system.

Due to fluctuations during the incident among conventional, contingency, and crisis care, and the categories (space, staff, supplies) that can be affected, it can become challenging at the regional level to keep this information current. It may be most relevant at the regional health care coalition level to keep track of capacity issues—examining whether hospitals are implementing crisis surge response care plans or whether EMS calls are being deferred. Consideration for keeping track of specific supply/staff issues in relation to requests for assistance may be most beneficially oriented toward specific lifesaving resources that are in short supply (e.g., ventilators).

The regional or coalition goal is to support transition and response to maintain enough balance in the system so that individual facilities/agencies are providing consistent levels of care, even though there may be daily and shift-based fluctuations across the system. The facility goal is to stay out of crisis care as much as possible—for example, a patient is triaged away from mechanical ventilation (crisis) due to lack of community resources, but if a ventilator is available at another facility the patient may be bag-valve ventilated during transfer there (contingency). If the patient is still alive when a ventilator becomes available, he/she would receive that "conventional" resource.

The state goal is to ensure that a consistent level of care and common decision-making strategies are provided in the jurisdiction, including identification of additional support, and coordinate with surrounding states to reduce interstate variability as much as possible. For noncontiguous states and territories, coordination with other states may not be feasible or considered high priority because they are far away, and assistance may take hours to arrive and prove logistically challenging. In certain situations (e.g., multistate incidents), however, aid may be most effectively sought from the state that suffered the least damage or has the most resources, or from other partners (e.g., Department of Defense [DoD] or private entities) rather than via usual adjacent partners. Planning discussions should reflect some of these variables.

Information Synthesis and Sharing

Key points: Information sharing and synthesis is critical to responding to a catastrophic disaster. Addressing potential barriers to the flow and movement of such information, both real and perceived, is a critical first step in preparing for the development and use of indicators and triggers needed to help guide the response to the implementation of crisis standards of care.

In the context of catastrophic disaster incidents—which, by their very definition, will entail local, regional, state, tribal, and federal response—the access to information and the ability to share such information across these jurisdictional domains will be critically important to a successful response. Although no surveillance system can ever be counted on to "make the diagnosis" in the case of a bioterror agent release, these systems will provide important situational awareness information and can help to develop the characteristics of an ongoing incident that will be very useful to the emergency response community. Examples of existing surveillance systems are discussed below. Addressing the potential barriers to the flow and movement of such information, both real and perceived, is a critical first step in preparing for the development and use of indicators and triggers needed to help guide the response to the implementation of crisis standards of care.

Important here is the recognition that a wide variety of information will be needed by the many elements of the emergency response system, not all of which will be accessible or available to all of the response disciplines. As discussed in Chapter 1, emergency management is in an excellent position to coordinate efforts of EMS, hospitals, and public health using the Emergency Support Function (ESF)-8 framework. Efforts to synthesize the available information, using the emergency management–led jurisdictional EOC, along with the use of a medical information clearinghouse concept, will be of significant value. For example, stressors emanating from one single incident may be seen across the entirety of the emergency response system. Taken alone, this information may not be as meaningful. A law enforcement concern about increasing civil unrest may come into focus only after it is recognized that there is a disease outbreak in one particular demographic group, leading to subtle but important population-based behavioral expressions of concern. The synthesis of such information will be most evident in communities that employ the use of multiagency coordination (MAC), which is "a process that allows all levels of government and all disciplines to work together more efficiently and effectively," often implemented using a Multiagency Coordination System (FEMA, 2013b).

Examples of Existing Data-Sharing Systems

Key point: Existing data sources and data-sharing systems can be leveraged for the development and use of indicators and triggers.

Many data-sharing systems have been developed and implemented by state and federal governments to help ensure prompt detection of incidents and aid in decision making and resource allocation during large-scale public health emergencies. These data-sharing systems may provide information that is useful for the development of indicators and triggers. In developing indicators and triggers for their communities, stakeholders should consider existing data-sharing systems and how they may be leveraged to guide decision making about transitions along the continuum of care. Select examples are discussed below. With regard to indicators and triggers in state and local CSC plans, most jurisdictions have yet to address this or are in relatively early stages; details are provided in Box 2-5.

It was beyond the scope of this report to comprehensively examine the benefits, limitations, and resource requirements of biosurveillance and other situational awareness systems. HHS is currently undertaking activities to develop a Public Health and Health Care Situational Awareness Strategy and Implementation Plan (Lurie, 2012). The National Biodefense Science Board reviewed the draft plan and provided guiding principles and recommendations aimed at improving public health and health care situational awareness, including emphasizing the need to "assure compatibility, consistency, continuity, coordination, and integration of all the disparate systems and data requirements" (NBSB, 2013, p. 3). An overview of existing public health surveillance, with an emphasis on the detection of bioterrorism threats, is available in an earlier Institute of Medicine (IOM) report (IOM and NRC, 2011).

Systems for Sharing Information About Prehospital and Hospital Resource Availability

The state of Maryland's Emergency Medical Resource Center is one of the first examples of a systematic approach to coordinating prehospital EMS and hospital response efforts, for daily use as well as in disaster incidents. In the aftermath of 9/11, a facility resource tracking system was put in place, coordinating information related to key data points, including bed availability, resource availability, staffing, and related issues (MIEMSS, 2013). Other state programs include those in New York, which created the Health Emergency Response Data System (Gotham et al., 2007). Like the Maryland system, this is a statewide electronic Web-based data collection system linking health care facilities, including all hospitals. This serves as the primary means for relaying resource requests to the State Department of Health, and can also be used to distribute just-in-time information, as well as serve as a tool to conduct rapid assessment surveys. These are two examples of statewide information management systems. Many more states have developed, or are developing, similar efforts, particularly as federal grant guidance highlights the importance of establishing situational awareness, including data sharing and analysis.

At the federal level, HAvBED was created under a contract from the Agency for Healthcare Research and Quality to help develop a national hospital bed reporting system that could be used to provide situational awareness of hospital bed availability during times of surge demand in care (AHRQ, 2005). It was born partly out of the experience of the Commonwealth of Virginia's early adoption of bed reporting capabilities that were in place and fully functional prior to the 9/11 attacks and the anthrax bioterror mailings. Like the early Maryland and New York state efforts, the Northern Virginia hospitals, not yet coalesced under the auspices of the regional coalition that was formed in 2002, had been using an Internet-based bed reporting system since 1999.[2] When the other regions in the state chose to implement a similar capability beginning in 2003, it was decided that the vendors would be asked to work together to ensure uniformity of reporting standards and data elements for this statewide system. The Northern Virginia hospitals continued to use the proprietary system that they had previously contracted to use, while the remaining five hospital regions chose a different vendor. The genesis of the HAvBED project was to ensure that open standards were used to allow for interoperability of data exchange, despite the selection of proprietary systems. The reporting of "bed availability" information remains an important marker of the general state of hospital readiness to absorb large numbers of potential casualties. Despite the numerous shortcomings of the reported data (may not reflect accurate numbers; often do not account for concurrent availability of staffing and resources to support the care of patients who might need those beds; and are dynamic values that can change faster than the numbers can be reported), this marker represents an "indicator" that is often taken to reflect basic health care system capacity and capability.

Another important limitation in our ability to achieve a common operating picture, particularly in the realm of the health care response to large-scale incidents, are the many barriers that exist to sharing patient information and tracking patients through the continuum of care—clinical outcomes, treatment modalities, and lessons learned—in near real time during large-scale medical emergencies. There is no good mechanism in place to allow for sharing of clinical information, particularly in the immediate context of an ongoing incident. Some local and regional information sharing may occur: for example, the use of informal networks of health care systems and providers during the anthrax attacks in 2001 permitted real-time exchange of information by providers who managed the anthrax cases with those in the surrounding communities who were concerned that more cases were going undiagnosed. This approach resulted in the successful diagnosis and treatment of the fifth of five inhalational anthrax cases identified in the Washington, DC, region (Gursky et al., 2003; Hanfling, 2011). However, in the setting of a larger-scale incident, it is imperative that there be a clearinghouse for case reports and clinical information exchange, as well as an expedited process for conducting intraincident research on the use of specific medical countermeasures or other treatment modalities that may be useful in improving the medical outcomes and decreasing morbidity and mortality.

Biosurveillance

ESSENCE is a biosurveillance system that was originally developed for the DoD to account for syndromic surveillance oriented toward the evaluation of emerging infectious disease agents across the globe (Lombardo et al., 2004). An updated version of this program was adopted by state and local governments in the Washington, DC, region for use by their public health agencies to help identify similar issues, including the release of potential bioterror agents in the community. Sharing agreements and protocols for data access were developed in order to effect the implementation of this system. In the case of the DC region, the primary flow of data is often oriented toward state public health departments, with intermittent sharing of data interpretation and analysis. However, this occurs in a cumbersome fashion, with most reports directed to local public health departments, not the hospitals from where the data are initially gathered.

The state of Michigan has had a biosurveillance system in place that serves as an example of how information from such systems can be shared more easily. The Michigan Syndromic Surveillance System

---

[2] Unpublished work; information from committee co-chair Dan Hanfling.

BOX 2-5
Examples and Analysis of Indicators and Triggers in Existing CSC Plans

In a 2012 report on the allocation of scarce resources during mass casualty events, it was noted that few state plans contained "operational frameworks for shifting to crisis standards of care" (Timbie et al., 2012, p. ES-9). The committee searched for and compiled 18 available jurisdictional plans that discussed triggers for crisis care or pandemic influenza.[1-18] Six of these discussed lab or World Health Organization criteria-based triggers for pandemic influenza and not relevant to crisis care.[6-8,11-12,16] A few states included state declarations of emergency as the trigger for increased information sharing and coordination, but not for triage.[1,4] One state referenced "unusual events" rather than triggers, which prompt enhanced information exchange within the system.[2] These were defined as events that significantly impact or threaten public health, environmental health, or medical services; are projected to require resources from outside the region; are politically sensitive or of high visibility; or otherwise require enhanced information exchange between partners or the state.

One state approached the "trigger" for crisis care from a process standpoint—that if a facility did not have a resource, could not get it, and could not transfer the patient, the situation met preexisting criteria for crisis care and resource allocation.[18] These preexisting criteria have been described in prior work by the IOM and the American College of Chest Physicians and should be incorporated in the decision-making process, if not in the trigger.[19-20]

The advantage of this approach is that it offers an all-inclusive process for resource shortfalls. The disadvantage to be considered is that, due to lack of specificity, it may result in less proactive decision making or anticipation of potential trigger events. This is a common trade-off with indicators and triggers—the less specific, the easier the development, but the less sensitive and less specific to the response. The more specific the indicators and triggers, the harder the development work, but with potentially improved system performance.

Other states and entities identified factors that were considered as "triggers" for resource triage, though these were categorical rather than specific aside from a specific staffing threshold in two plans (which may be more relevant to certain job classes or facilities of certain size—no validation of these numbers or references were noted; using expert-based indicators and triggers is the current state of the science, and a systematic approach to evaluation would be useful).[1-2,4-5,10,13-15,17-18]

- Equipment shortages—including ventilators, beds, blood products, antivirals, antibiotics, operating room capacity, personal protective equipment (PPE), including supply chain disruption or recall/contamination, emergency medical services (EMS) units;
- Staff/personnel triggers—subspecialty staff, security, trauma team, EMS;
- Space triggers—unable to accommodate all patients requiring hospitalization despite maximal surge measures, doubling of patient rooms;
- Infrastructure—including loss of facilities, essential services, or isolation of a facility due to flooding or other access problems;
- Numbers of patients in excess of planned health care facility capacity, or an exceptional surge in number and severity over a short period of time;
- Use of alternate care facilities;
- Marked increase in proportion of patients who are critically ill and unlikely to survive;
- Abnormally high percentage of hospitals on divert for EMS;
- Increase in influenza hospitalizations and deaths reported or other surveillance or forecasting data suggesting surge in excess of resources;

- Marked increase in staff or school absenteeism (two specifying 20-30 percent or >30 percent thresholds);
- Increased emergency medical dispatch call volumes;
- Increased requests for mutual aid or activation of statewide mutual aid agreements;
- Depletion of state assets;
- Unavailability of assets from other states; and
- Depletion of federal assets.

Of note, one county's pandemic flu plan specified 30 elements of intensive care patient data gathering. Though the specific dataset elements have not been validated and potentially could be optimized, the gathering of clinical data in real time in order to provide aggregate information about severity of disease and treatment effect is a key gap in current national planning for infectious disease incidents.

Available plans tended to list indicators, for the most part without specific thresholds.[2-5,7,9,10,13-14,19] This is actually consistent with the fact that most of the plans were state level, and thus unlikely to identify indicators of sufficient certainty to establish triggers, aiming primarily to identify the key resources expected to be in shortage and potential indicators from available systems data or functional thresholds (alternate care site use, etc.) marking the transition to crisis care. This is likely to be as specific as state-level plans can be, though national planning should include guidance for shortages of antivirals, vaccine, or PPE, for which basic assumptions and triggers for policy and clinical guidance should be developed.

The types of indicators and triggers may be less specific at higher tiers, but should be linked to the actions that would be taken by each tier. At the state level, a lack of specificity is acceptable at the state level because much of the data is uncertain and requires analysis and a non-scripted response from state agencies. Triggers that may be appropriate at the state level (opening of alternate care sites) are unhelpful at the local level because they will occur too late to be of assistance in the early management of an escalating incident. Local triggers should be as concrete as possible and provide enough advance warning to take action, rather than only triggering when a crisis situation has already occurred (i.e., better to have an early scripted trigger for notification of an emergency management group to assess a situation rather than a late trigger when the system runs out of ventilators).

SOURCES
[1]Alaskan Health Care Providers and Medical Emergency Preparedness–Pediatrics (MEP-P) Project [draft], 2008.
[2]California Department of Public Health and California Emergency Medical Services Authority, 2011.
[3]City of Albuquerque, Office of Emergency Management, 2005.
[4]Colorado Department of Public Health and Environment, 2009.
[5]Florida Department of Health, 2011.
[6]Indiana State Department of Health, 2009.
[7]Kansas Department of Health and Environment, 2013.
[8]Kentucky Department of Public Health, Division of Epidemiology and Health Planning, Cabinet for Health and Family Services, 2007.
[9]King County, Seattle Health Care Coalition, and Northwest Healthcare Response Network, 2009.
[10]Minnesota Department of Health, Office of Emergency Preparedness, 2012.
[11]New Hampshire Department of Health and Human Services, 2007.
[12]New York State Department of Health, 2008.
[13]Northern Utah Healthcare Coalition, 2010.
[14]Ohio Department of Health and Ohio Hospital Association, 2012.
[15]State of Michigan, 2012b.
[16]Tennessee Department of Health, 2009.
[17]Utah Hospitals and Health Systems Association for the Utah Department of Health, 2009.
[18]Wisconsin Hospital Association, Inc., 2010.
[19]Devereaux et al., 2008.
[20]IOM, 2012a.

(MSSS) is "a real-time surveillance system that tracks chief presenting complaints from emergent care settings, enabling public health officials and providers to monitor trends and investigate unusual increases in symptom presentations" (State of Michigan, 2012a, 2013). Health care facilities have enrolled to participate voluntarily on an ongoing basis since the system was launched in 2003; currently, 89 facilities submit data electronically to the MSSS.[3] The system continues to evolve to support public health and information technology needs. In 2013, the MSSS will be able to receive data from health care professionals in settings other than hospital emergency departments, in support of Meaningful Use, which involves using electronic health record technology to ensure complete and accurate information, better access to information, and patient empowerment (CMS, 2013; HealthIT.gov, 2013). In 2012, the MSSS processed more than 4.3 million ED registrations. The chief complaints from ED registrations are categorized using a free-text complaint coder. Trends in the categorical groups are analyzed using an adaptive recursive least squares algorithm, and alerts are sent to Michigan public health officials when unusual increases in symptom presentations are detected. In addition, the MSSS supports enhanced surveillance that is conducted during high-profile events (e.g., local NCAA basketball tournament games, World Series, Super Bowl, and North American International Auto Show), with findings distributed to stakeholders. Access to the MSSS interface is role based: participating health care facilities can visualize and report on their own data, including the ability to run ad hoc queries. The local health departments can view data from within their jurisdictions, and key Michigan Department of Community Health staffs have full statewide access. Since 2008, MSSS data contributions have informed national influenza surveillance via the Distribute Project and national syndromic surveillance efforts via Biosense, soon to be resumed with the redesigned Biosense 2.0 (see CDC, 2012a).

The benefits and costs of creating new surveillance systems that are highly dependent on technology or labor for data entry should be carefully considered. For a discussion of the benefits, limitations, and resource requirements of syndromic surveillance, see IOM and NRC (2011).

Indicators and Triggers in U.S. Department of Veterans Affairs Medical Centers (VAMCs) and Military Treatment Facilities (MTFs)

The coordination of VAMCs and MTFs into planning efforts and response to catastrophic disaster events is of vital importance to the two constituencies served by these unique health care organizations. Both can be considered to be "closed" systems, focused on the delivery of care to specific patient populations that they are entrusted to serve: namely, veterans and active-duty military and their dependents. But both systems are also recognized to be important components of the local and regional health care communities in which they are located, particularly for a disaster response. At the local level, VAMC and MTF leadership are given the authorization to provide care to the communities in which they are situated, invoking principles of humanitarian assistance to ensure that patient care needs are addressed when the entire community is under duress. In the evolving efforts to better organize health care entities to respond to disaster events, VAMC and MTF facilities have been encouraged to become members of health care coalitions. For example, the Washington, DC, VAMC, the former Walter Reed Army Medical Center, and Bethesda National Naval Medical Center (now combined as the Walter Reed National Military Medical Center at Bethesda, Maryland) have been

---

[3] Unpublished work; information from committee member Linda Scott.

a central component of the DC Hospital Coalition. In Northern Virginia, DeWitt Army Hospital at Fort Belvoir was a founding member of the Northern Virginia Hospital Alliance.[4]

In this regard, the functions of VAMC and MTF facilities during disaster events are best considered to be component parts of the larger, regional health care system. Therefore, they will be expected to use similar indicators, triggers, and tactics as those used by their public- and private-sector counterparts. In the case of mature health care coalitions that have included these facilities within their membership, the use of situational awareness tools in place across the community are likely to provide this information to all member hospitals, including those in the Department of Veterans Affairs (VA) and DoD. In those communities in which the development of health care coalitions is still evolving, the VA and DoD facilities may be in position to help coordinate and facilitate the sharing of key information. This is particularly true given their connectivity to a network of information systems, supply chains, and health care facilities that are located outside of the immediate community, all part of a national health care system.

One of the difficulties that VAMC and MTF leadership may face under catastrophic response conditions will be determining how to parse available resources between two distinct mission profiles: service to their members and provision of care to the community at large. In this respect, there may be "internal" indicators specific to the VA or DoD system that will have to be evaluated in addition to those usual measures being used to determine local and regional capabilities. The community and the VA/DoD system may have different data needs and community and national systems indicators may vary, so the systems used to collect these may not be standardized. These facilities walk a fine line in a crisis situation, as it is not to anyone's best interest if the level of care provided at the institution is inconsistent with that being provided in the community, but these are not "community facilities." For example, VA facilities may have substantially more burdens than community hospitals during influenza epidemics affecting the elderly, while military facilities have substantially less; balancing these demands against a local coalition's resources may be very helpful in easing strain on the system, and proactive ways to accomplish this should be explored with the facilities (e.g., a local VA might prefer to accept those with prior service connections in preference to non-selected patients during a community crisis). Consideration of CSC planning by leadership located at the Veterans Integrated Service Network level, Veterans Health Administration, and Defense Health Headquarters (DoD) will be crucial to the successful implementation of the tactics derived from the analysis of key indicators.

Legal Indicators and Triggers

Detailed examination of legal issues is outside of the scope of this project, although there may be interesting issues regarding legal indicators and triggers that deserve additional attention (see Box 2-6[5]). For more discussion and details about the ethical principles and legal issues, see the Institute of Medicine's previous reports on crisis standards of care (IOM, 2009, 2012a).

---

[4] Unpublished work; information from committee co-chair Dan Hanfling.
[5] The committee would like to thank James Hodge of Arizona State University for his comments on the material in Box 2-6.

SUMMARY

In planning, facilities and agencies should first identify the key response strategies they will use. Second, data sources and information that inform these thresholds should be examined and optimized. Third, actions to be taken when the trigger is reached should be determined; are they scripted or non-scripted? Fourth, are there scripted tactics that can be employed, or should the tactics be non-scripted and incident-specific?

Determination of indicators and triggers can seem daunting. However, discussing these issues at all tiers of the emergency response system will help clarify and develop indicators and triggers that will inform decision making and help deliver the best possible care during a disaster, given the circumstances. The toolkit in the subsequent chapters will facilitate these conversations.

REFERENCES

AHRQ (Agency for Healthcare Research and Quality). 2005. *National hospital available beds for emergencies and disasters (HAvBED) System*. Rockville, MD: AHRQ. http://archive.ahrq.gov/prep/havbed/index.html (accessed April 13, 2013).

Alaskan Health Care Providers and Medical Emergency Preparedness-Pediatrics (MEP-P) Project. 2008 [draft]. *Medical Alaskan technical recommendations for pediatric medical triage and resource allocation in a disaster*. Alaskan Health Care Providers and Medical Emergency Preparedness-Pediatrics (MEP-P) Project. http://a2p2.com/oldsite/mep-p/ethics/MEP-P_Technical_Recommendations_with_Appendices_DRAFT_7-08.PDF (accessed February 14, 2013).

Asplin, B. R., T. J. Flottemesch, and B. D. Gordon. 2006. Developing models for patient flow and daily surge capacity research. *Academic Emergency Medicine* 13(11):1109-1113.

ASPR (Assistant Secretary for Preparedness and Response). 2013. *MedMap*. Washington, DC: Department of Health and Human Services. https://medmap.hhs.gov (accessed April 3, 2013).

Barbisch, D. F., and K. L. Koenig. 2006. Understanding surge capacity: Essential elements. *Academic Emergency Medicine* 13(11):1098-1102.

Bayram, J. D., and S. Zuabi. 2012. Disaster metrics: Quantification of acute medical disasters in trauma related multiple casualty events through modeling of the Acute Medical Severity Index. *Prehospital and Disaster Medicine* 27(2):130-135.

Bayram, J. D., S. Zuabi, and I. Subbarao. 2011. Disaster metrics: Quantitative benchmarking of hospital surge capacity in trauma-related multiple casualty incidents. *Disaster Medicine and Public Health Preparedness* 5(2):117-124.

Bayram, J. D., S. Zuabi, and M.J. Sayed. 2012. Disaster metrics: Quantitative estimation of the number of ambulances required in trauma-related multiple casualty events. *Prehospital and Disaster Medicine* 27(5):445-451.

Bradt, D. A., P. Aitken, G. Fitzgerald, R. Swift, G. O'Reilly, and B. Bartley. 2009. Emergency department surge capacity: Recommendations of the Australasian Surge Strategy Working Group. *Academic Emergency Management* 16(12):1350-1358.

Brownstein, J. S., C. C. Freifeld, and L. C. Madoff. 2009. Digital disease detection—harnessing the Web for public health surveillance. *New England Journal of Medicine* 360(21):2153-2157.

Buehler, J. W., A. Sonricker, M. Paladini, P. Soper, and F. Mostashari. 2008. Syndromic surveillance practice in the United States: Findings from a survey of state, territorial, and selected local health departments. *Advances in Disease Surveillance* 6(3):1-20. http://www.isdsjournal.org/articles/2618.pdf (accessed June 11, 2013).

Buehler, J. W., E. A. Whitney, D. Smith, M. J. Prietula, S. H. Stanton, and A. P. Isakov. 2009. Situational uses of syndromic surveillance. *Biosecurity and Bioterrorism: Biodefense Strategy, Practice, and Science* 7(2):165-177.

Burkle, F.M., E. B. Hsu, M. Loehr, M. D. Christian, D. Markenson, L. Rubinson, and F. L. Archer. 2007. Definition and functions of Health Unified Command and Emergency Operations Centers for large-scale bioevent disasters within the existing ICS. *Disaster Medicine and Public Health Preparedness* 1(2):135-141.

Butler, D. 2013. When Google got flu wrong. *Nature* 494(7436):155-156.

California Department of Public Health and California Emergency Medical Services Authority. 2011. *California public health and medical emergency operations manual*. http://www.emsa.ca.gov/disaster/files/EOM712011.pdf (accessed February 14, 2013).

Carneiro, H. A., and E. Mylonakis. 2009. Google trends: A Web-based tool for real-time surveillance of disease outbreaks. *Clinical Infectious Diseases* 49(10):1557-1564.

CDC (Centers for Disease Control and Prevention). 2003. *Mass casualties predictor*. Atlanta, GA: CDC. http://www.bt.cdc.gov/masscasualties/predictor.asp (accessed March 11, 2013).

CDC. 2010. *Blast injuries: Fact sheets for professionals*. Atlanta, GA: CDC. http://www.bt.cdc.gov/masscasualties/pdf/blast_fact_sheet_professionals-a.pdf (accessed March 10, 2013).

CDC. 2012a. *BioSense program*. Atlanta, GA: CDC. http://www.cdc.gov/biosense (accessed June 10, 2013).

CDC. 2012b. *Overview of influenza surveillance in the United States*. Atlanta, GA: CDC. http://www.cdc.gov/flu/pdf/weekly/overview.pdf (accessed March 5, 2013).

CDC. 2013. *FluView: 2012-2013 Influenza season week 14 ending April 6, 2013*. Atlanta, GA: CDC. http://www.cdc.gov/flu/weekly (accessed March 5, 2013).

Challen, K., and D. Walter. 2006. Accelerated discharge of patients in the event of a major incident: Observational study of a teaching hospital. *BMC Public Health* 6(1):108.

City of Albuquerque, Office of Emergency Management. 2005. *A strategic guide for the city-wide response to and recovery from major emergencies and disasters (Annex 6—health and medical)*. Albuquerque, NM: City of Albuquerque, Office of Emergency Management. http://www.cabq.gov/police/emergency-management-office/documents/Annex6Healthand Medical.pdf (accessed February 14, 2013).

City of Boston. 2013 (January 9). Mayor Menino declares public health emergency as flu epidemic worsens. http://www. cityofboston.gov/news/Default.aspx?id=5922 (accessed March 11, 2013).

CMS (Centers for Medicare & Medicaid Services). 2013. *Meaningful use*. Baltimore, MD: CMS. http://www.cms.gov/ Regulations-and-Guidance/Legislation/EHRIncentivePrograms/Meaningful_Use.html (accessed May 3, 2013).

Colorado Department of Public Health and Environment. 2009. *Guidance for alterations in the healthcare system during moderate to severe influenza pandemic*. Denver, CO: Colorado Department of Public Health and Environment.

Cook, S., C. Conrad, A. L. Fowlkes, and M. H. Mohebbi. 2011. Assessing Google Flu Trends performance in the United States during the 2009 influenza virus A (H1N1) pandemic. *PLoS ONE* 6(8):e23510.

Davidson, S. J., K. L. Koenig, and D. C. Cone. 2006. Daily patient flow is not surge: Management is prediction. *Academic Emergency Medicine* 13(11):1095-1096.

de Boer, J. 1999. Order in chaos: Modeling medical management in disasters. *European Journal of Emergency Medicine* 6(2):141-148.

DeLia, D. 2006. Annual bed statistics give a misleading picture of hospital surge capacity. *Annals of Emergency Medicine* 48(4):384-388.

Devereaux, A. V., J. R. Dichter, M. D. Christian, N. N. Dubler, C. E. Sandrock, J. L. Hick, T. Powell, J. A. Geiling, D. E. Amundson, T. E. Baudendistel, D. A. Braner, M. A. Klein, K. A. Berkowitz, J.R. Curtis, and L. Rubinson. 2008. Definitive care for the critically ill during a disaster: A framework for allocation of scarce resources in mass critical care. From a Task Force for Mass Critical Care summit meeting, January 26-27, 2007, Chicago, IL. *Chest* 133(Suppl 5):S51-S66. http://www.ceep.ca/resources/Definitive-Care-Critically-Ill-Disaster.pdf (accessed March 4, 2013).

Dugas, A. F., Y. H. Hsieh, S. R. Levin, J. M. Pines, D. P. Mareiniss, A. Mohareb, C. A. Gaydos, T. M. Perl, and R. E. Rothman. 2012. Google Flu Trends: Correlated with emergency department influenza rates and crowding metrics. *Clinical Infectious Diseases* 54(4):463-469.

Dugas, A. F., M. Jalalpour, Y. Gel, S. Levin, F. Torcaso, and T. Igusa. 2013. Influenza forecasting with Google Flu Trends. *PLoS ONE* 8(2):e56176.

EMSA (California Emergency Medical Services Authority). 2007. *Disaster Medical Services Division—Hospital Incident Command System (HICS)*. http://www.emsa.ca.gov/hics (accessed March 11, 2013).

Espino, J., W. Hogan, and M. Wagner. 2003. Telephone triage: A timely data source for surveillance of influenza-like diseases. *AMIA Annual Symposium Proceedings* 2003:215-219.

FEMA (Federal Emergency Management Agency). 2013a. *National Incident Management System (NIMS)*. http://www.fema. gov/emergency/nims (accessed March 11, 2013).

FEMA. 2013b. *Multiagency coordination systems*. http://www.fema.gov/multiagency-coordination-systems (accessed May 15, 2013).

Florida Department of Health. 2011 (April 5). *Pandemic influenza: Triage and scarce resource allocation guidelines*. Tallahassee: Florida Department of Health. http://www.doh.state.fl.us/demo/bpr/PDFs/ACS-GUIDE-Ver10-5.pdf (accessed February 14, 2013).

Flu Near You. 2013. *Flu near you*. https://flunearyou.org (accessed March 5, 2013).

Furbee, P. M., J. H. Coben, S. K. Smyth, W. G. Manley, D. E. Summers, N. D. Sanddal, T. L. Sanddal, J. C. Helmkamp, R. L. Kimble, R. C. Althouse, and A. T. Kocsis. 2006. Realities of rural emergency medical services disaster preparedness. *Prehospital Disaster Medicine* 21(2):64-70.

Garrett, L. 2009 (June 12). Interview. *Hurdles in declaring swine flu a pandemic*. Council on Foreign Relations. http://www.cfr. org/public-health-threats/hurdles-declaring-swine-flu-pandemic/p19617 (accessed March 11, 2013).

GFT (Google Flu Trends). 2013. *Google flu trends*. http://www.google.org/flutrends (accessed March 5, 2013).

Ginsberg, J., M. H. Mohebbi, R. S. Patel, L. Brammer, M. S. Smolinksi, and L. Brilliant. 2009. Detecting influenza epidemics using search engine query data. *Nature* 457(7232):1012-1014.

Gotham, I. J., D. L. Sottolano, M. E. Hennessy, J. P. Napoli, G. Dobkins, L. H. Le, R. H. Burhans, and B. I. Fage. 2007. An integrated information system for all-hazards health preparedness and response: New York State Health Emergency Response Data System. *Journal of Public Health Management and Practice* 13(5):486-496.

Gursky, E., T. V. Inglesby, and T. O'Toole. 2003. Anthrax 2001: Observations on the medical and public health response. *Biosecurity and Bioterrorism* 1(2):97-110.

Handler, J. A., M. Gillam, T. D. Kirsch, and C. F. Feied. 2006. Metrics in the science of surge. *Academic Emergency Medicine* 13(11):1173-1178.

Hanfling, D. 2011. Public health response to terrorism and bioterrorism: Inventing the wheel. In *Remembering 9/11 and anthrax: Public health's role in national defense*. Washington, DC: Trust for America's Health. http://healthyamericans.org/assets/files/TFAH911Anthrax10YrAnnvFINAL.pdf (accessed May 3, 2013).

HealthIT.gov. 2013. *Meaningful use*. http://www.healthit.gov/policy-researchers-implementers/meaningful-use (accessed May 15, 2013).

HealthMap. 2013. *HealthMap*. http://healthmap.org/en (accessed April 3, 2013).

Hick, J. L., K. L. Koenig, D. Barbisch, and T. A. Bey. 2008. Surge capacity concepts for health care facilities: The CO-S-TR model for initial incident assessment. *Disaster Medicine and Public Health Preparedness* 2(Suppl 1):S51-S57.

Hirschberg, A., G. S. Bradford, T. Granchi, M. J. Wall, K. L. Mattox, and M. Stein. 2005. How does casualty load affect trauma care in urban bombing incidents? A quantitative analysis. *Journal of Trauma* 58(4):686-695.

Indiana State Department of Health. 2009. *Pandemic influenza outbreak plan*. Indianapolis, IN: Indiana State Department of Health. http://www.state.in.us/isdh/files/PandemicInfluenzaPlan.pdf (accessed February 14, 2013).

IOM (Institute of Medicine). 2007a. *Emergency medical services: At the crossroads*. Washington, DC: The National Academies Press. http://www.nap.edu/catalog.php?record_id=11629 (accessed June 7, 2013).

IOM. 2007b. *Hospital-based emergency care: At the breaking point*. Washington, DC: The National Academies Press. http://www.nap.edu/catalog.php?record_id=11621 (accessed June 7, 2013).

IOM. 2009. *Guidance for establishing crisis standards of care for use in disaster situations: A letter report*. Washington, DC: The National Academies Press. http://www.nap.edu/catalog.php?record_id=12749 (accessed April 3, 2013).

IOM. 2012a. *Crisis standards of care: A systems framework for catastrophic disaster response*. Washington, DC: The National Academies Press. http://www.nap.edu/openbook.php?record_id=13351 (accessed April 3, 2013).

IOM. 2012b. *Public engagement on facilitating access to antiviral medications and information in an influenza pandemic: Workshop series summary*. Washington, DC: The National Academies Press. http://www.nap.edu/catalog.php?record_id=13404 (accessed May 31, 2013).

IOM and NRC (National Research Council). 2011. *BioWatch and public health surveillance: Evaluating systems for the early detection of biological threats. Abbreviated version*. Washington, DC: The National Academies Press. http://www.nap.edu/catalog.php?record_id=12688 (accessed June 7, 2013).

Israel Ministry of Health. 1976. *Sahar Committee for Hospital Preparedness*. Tel Aviv: Israel Ministry of Health.

Jenkins, J. L., R. E. O'Connor, and D. C. Cone. 2006. Differentiating large-scale surge versus daily surge. *Academic Emergency Medicine* 13(11):1169-1172.

Kaji, A., K. L. Koenig, and T. Bey. 2006. Surge capacity for healthcare systems: A conceptual framework. *Academic Emergency Medicine* 13(11):1157–1159.

Kansas Department of Health and Environment. 2013. *Kansas pandemic influenza preparedness and response plan*. Topeka: Kansas Department of Health and Environment. http://www.kdheks.gov/cphp/download/KS_PF_Plan.pdf (accessed February 14, 2013).

Kanter, R. K. 2007. Strategies to improve pediatric disaster surge response: Potential mortality reduction and tradeoffs. *Critical Care Medicine* 35(12):2837-2842.

Kelen, G. D., C. K. Kraus, M. L. McCarthy, E. Bass, E. B. Hsu, G. Li, J. J. Scheulen, J. B. Shahan, J. D. Brill, and G. B. Green. 2006. Inpatient disposition classification for the creation of hospital surge capacity: A multiphase study. *Lancet* 368(9551):1984-1990.

Kelen, G. D., M. L. McCarthy, C. K. Kraus, R. Ding, E. B. Hsu, G. Li, J. B. Shahan, J. J. Scheulen, and G. B. Green. 2009. Creation of surge capacity by early discharge of hospitalized patients at low risk for untoward events. *Disaster Medicine and Public Health Preparedness* 3(Suppl 2):S10-S16.

Kellermann, A. L., A. P. Isakov, R. Parker, M. T. Handrigan, and S. Foldy. 2010. Web-based self-triage of influenza-like illness during the 2009 H1N1 influenza pandemic. *Annals of Emergency Medicine* 56(3):288-294.

Kentucky Department of Public Health, Division of Epidemiology and Health Planning. 2007. *Kentucky pandemic influenza preparedness plan*. Frankfort: Kentucky Department of Public Health, Division of Epidemiology and Health Planning. http://chfs.ky.gov/nr/rdonlyres/6cd366d2-6726-4ad0-85bb-e83cf769560e/0/kypandemicinfluenzapreparednessplan.pdf (accessed February 14, 2013).

King County, Seattle Health Care Coalition, and Northwest Healthcare Response Network. 2009 (unpublished). *H1N1 ICU data questions*.

Kirsch, T., L. Sauer, and D. Guha Sapir. 2012. Analysis of the international and US response to the Haiti earthquake: Recommendations for change. *Disaster Medicine and Public Health Preparedness* 6(3):200-208.

Koonin, L. M., and D. Hanfling. 2013. Broadening access to medical care during a severe influenza pandemic: The CDC nurse triage line project. *Biosecurity and Bioterrorism: Biodefense Strategy, Practice, and Science* 11(1):75-80.

Kosashvili, Y., L. Aharonson-Daniel, K. Peleg, A. Horowitz, D. Laor, and A. Blumenfeld. 2009. Israeli hospital preparedness for terrorism-related multiple casualty incidents: Can the surge capacity and injury severity distribution be better predicted? *Injury* 40(7):727-731.

Lombardo, J. S., H. Burkom, and J. Pavlin. 2004. Essence II and the framework for evaluating syndromic surveillance systems. *Morbidity and Mortality Weekly Report* 53(Suppl):159-165.

Lurie, N. 2012 (June 7). *Nicole Lurie to John Parker and members of the National Biodefense Science Board (NBSB)*. Letter. Washington, DC: ASPR. http://www.phe.gov/Preparedness/legal/boards/nbsb/Documents/sa-evaluation.pdf (accessed June 10, 2013).

Magruder, S. F., S. H. Lewis, A. Najmi, and E. Florio. 2004. Progress in understanding and using over-the-counter pharmaceuticals for syndromic surveillance. *Mortality and Morbidity Weekly Report* 53(Suppl):117-122.

Manley, W. G., P. M. Furbee, J. H. Coben, S. K. Smyth, D. E. Summers, R. C. Althourse, R. L. Kimble, A. T. Kocsis, and J. C. Helmkamp. 2006. Realities of disaster preparedness in rural hospitals. *Disaster Management and Response* 4(3):80-87.

MappyHealth. 2013. *MappyHealth*. http://mappyhealth.com (accessed March 5, 2013).

McCarthy, M. L., D. Aronsky, and G. D. Kelen. 2006. The measurement of daily surge and its relevance to disaster preparedness. *Academic Emergency Medicine* 13(11):1138-1141.

McCarthy, M. L., S. L. Zeger, R. Ding, D. Aronsky, N. R. Hoot, and G. D. Kelen. 2008. The challenge of predicting demand for emergency department services. *Academic Emergency Medicine* 15(4):337-346.

Merriam-Webster Dictionary. 2013. *Definition of "threshold."* Springfield, MA: Encyclopaedia Britannica. http://www.merriam-webster.com/dictionary/threshold (accessed April 3, 2013).

MIEMSS (Maryland Institute for Emergency Medical Services Systems). 2013. *EMRC/SYSCOM*. http://www.miemss.org/home/Departments/EMRCSYSCOM/tabid/139/Default.aspx (accessed February 1, 2013).

Minnesota Department of Health, Office of Emergency Preparedness. 2012. *Minnesota healthcare system preparedness program*. St. Paul: Minnesota Department of Health, Office of Emergency Preparedness. http://www.publichealthpractices.org/sites/cidrappractices.org/files/upload/372/372_protocol.pdf (accessed February 14, 2013).

NBSB (National Biodefense Science Board). 2013. *An evaluation of our nation's public health and healthcare situational awareness: A brief report from the National Biodefense Science Board (NBSB)*. Washington, DC: ASPR. http://www.phe.gov/Preparedness/legal/boards/nbsb/Documents/sa-evaluation.pdf (accessed June 10, 2013).

New Hampshire Department of Health and Human Services. 2007. *Influenza pandemic public health preparedness and response*. Concord: New Hampshire Department of Health and Human Services. http://www.dhhs.state.nh.us/dphs/cdcs/avian/documents/pandemic-plan.pdf (accessed February 14, 2013).

New York State Department of Health. 2008. *Pandemic influenza plan*. Albany: New York State Department of Health. http://www.health.ny.gov/diseases/communicable/influenza/pandemic/plan/docs/pandemic_influenza_plan.pdf (accessed February 14, 2013).

Northern Utah Healthcare Coalition. 2010. *Northern Utah regional medical surge capacity plan*. http://www.brhd.org/index.php?option=com_content&task=view&id=457&Itemid=31 (accessed February 14, 2013).

Ohio Department of Health and Ohio Hospital Association. 2012 [draft]. *Ohio medical coordination plan*: Emergency medical service annex. Columbus: Ohio Department of Health.

Ortiz, J. R., H. Zhou, D. K. Shay, K. M. Neuzil, A. L. Fowlkes, and C. H. Goss. 2011. Monitoring influenza activity in the United States: A comparison of traditional surveillance systems with Google Flu Trends. *PLoS ONE* 6(4):e18687.

Peleg, K., and A. L. Kellermann. 2009. Enhancing hospital surge capacity for mass casualty events. *Journal of the American Medical Association* 302(5):565-567.

Perry, A. G., K. M. Moore, L. E. Levesque, W. L. Pickett, and M. J. Korenberg. 2010. A comparison of methods for forecasting emergency department visits for respiratory illness using Telehealth Ontario calls. *Canadian Journal of Public Health* 101(6):464-469.

Polgreen, P. M., Y. Chen, D. M. Pennock, F. D. Nelson, and R. A. Weinstein. 2008. Using Internet searches for influenza surveillance. *Clinical Infectious Diseases* 47(11):1443-1448.

Price, R. A., D. Fagbuyi, R. Harris, D. Hanfling, F. Place, T. B. Todd, and A. L. Kellermann. 2013. Feasibility of web-based self-triage by parents of children with influenza-like illness: A cautionary tale. *Journal of the American Medical Association Pediatrics* 167(2):112-118.

Rivara, F. P., A. B. Nathens, G. J. Jurkovich, and R. V. Maier. 2006. Do trauma centers have the capacity to respond to disasters? *Journal of Trauma* 61(4):949-953.

Rolland, E., K. Moore, V. A. Robinson, and D. McGuiness. 2006. Using Ontario's "telehealth" health telephone helpline as an early-warning system: A study protocol. *BMC Health Services Research* 6:10-16.

Satterthwaite, P. S., and C. J. Atkinson. 2012. Using "reverse triage" to create hospital surge capacity: Royal Darwin Hospital's response to the Ashmore Reef disaster. *Emergency Medicine Journal* 29(2):160-162.

Schmidt, C. W. 2012. Using social media to predict and track disease outbreaks. *Environmental Health Perspectives* 120(1):A31-A33.

Schull, M. J. 2006. Hospital surge capacity: If you can't always get what you want, can you get what you need? *Annals Emergency Medicine* 48(4):389-390.

Schweigler, L. M., J. S. Desmond, M. L. McCarthy, K. J. Bukowski, E. L. Ionides, and J. G. Younger. 2009. Forecasting models of emergency department crowding. *Academic Emergency Medicine* 16(4):301-308.

Sickweather. 2013. *Sickweather.* http://www.sickweather.com (accessed March 5, 2013).

Signorini, A., A. M. Segre, and P. M. Polgreen. 2011. The use of Twitter to track levels of disease activity and public concern in the U.S. during the Influenza A H1N1 pandemic. *PLoS ONE* 6(5):e19467.

Sprung, C. L., J. L. Zimmerman, M. D. Christian, G. M. Joynt, J. L. Hick, B. Taylor, G. A. Richards, C. Sandrock, R. Cohen, and B. Adini. 2010. Recommendations for intensive care unit and hospital preparations for an influenza epidemic or mass disaster: Summary report of the European Society of Intensive Care Medicine's Task Force for intensive care unit triage during an influenza epidemic or mass disaster. *Intensive Care Medicine* 36(3):428-443.

State of Michigan. 2012a. *The Michigan Syndromic Surveillance System (MSSS)—Electronic syndromic submission to the Michigan Department of Community Health: Background and electronic syndromic surveillance reporting detail for MSSS.* Lansing, MI: Department of Community Health. http://michiganhit.org/docs/Syndromic%20Submission%20Guide.pdf (accessed May 21, 2013).

State of Michigan. 2012b. *Guidelines for Ethical Allocation of Scarce Medical Resources and Services during Public Health Emergencies in Michigan.* Lansing, MI: Department of Community Health, Office of Public Health Preparedness. http://www.mymedicalethics.net/Documentation/Michigan%20DCH%20Ethical%20Scarce%20Resources%20Guidelines%20v.2.0%20rev.%20Nov%202012%20Guidelines%20Only.pdf (accessed February 14, 2013).

State of Michigan. 2013. *Michigan Emergency Department Syndromic Surveillance System.* Lansing, MI: Department of Community Health. http://www.michigan.gov/mdch/0,4612,7-132-2945_5104_31274-107091--,00.html (accessed April 12, 2013).

State of New York Executive Chamber. 2013 (January 12). Declaring a disaster emergency in the state of New York and temporarily authorizing pharmacists to immunize children against seasonal influenza. http://www.governor.ny.gov/executive order/90 (accessed March 11, 2013).

Subbarao, I., M. K. Wynia, and F. M. Burkle. 2010. The elephant in the room: Collaboration and competition among relief organizations during high-profile disasters. *Journal of Clinical Ethics* 21(4):328-334.

Tadmor, B., J. McManus, and K. L. Koenig. 2006. The art and science of surge: Experience from Israel and the U.S. military. *Academic Emergency Medicine* 13(11):1130-1134.

Tennessee Department of Health. 2009. *Pandemic influenza response plan.* Nashville: Tennessee Department of Health. http://health.state.tn.us/ceds/PDFs/2006_PanFlu_Plan.pdf (accessed February 14, 2013).

Timbie, J. W., J. S. Ringel, D. S. Fox, D. A. Waxman, F. Pillemer, C. Carey, M. Moore, V. Karir, T. J. Johnson, N. Iyer, J. Hu, R. Shanman, J. W. Larkin, M. Timmer, A. Motala, T. R. Perry, S. Newberry, and A. L. Kellermann. 2012. *Allocation of scarce resources during mass casualty events.* Rockville, MD: AHRQ. http://www.ncbi.nlm.nih.gov/books/NBK98854/pdf/TOC.pdf (accessed June 6, 2013).

Utah Hospitals and Health Systems Association for the Utah Department of Health. 2009. *Utah pandemic influenza hospital and ICU triage guidelines.* Salt Lake City: Utah Hospitals and Health Systems Association for the Utah Department of Health. http://pandemicflu.utah.gov/plan/med_triage081109.pdf (accessed February 14, 2013).

van Dijk, A., D. McGuiness, E. Rolland, and K. M. Moore. 2008. Can Telehealth Ontario respiratory call volume be used as a proxy for emergency department respiratory visit surveillance by public health? *Canadian Journal of Emergency Medicine* 10(1):18-24.

WHO (World Health Organization). 2011. *Strengthening response to pandemics and other public-health emergencies. Report of the review committee on the functioning of the international health regulations (2005) and on pandemic influenza (H1N1) 2009.* Geneva, Switzerland: WHO. http://www.who.int/ihr/publications/RC_report/en/index.html (accessed March 11, 2013).

Wiler, J. L., R. T. Griffey, and T. Olsen. 2011. Review of modeling approaches for emergency department patient flow and crowding research. *Academic Emergency Medicine* 18(12):1371-1379.

Wisconsin Hospital Association, Inc. 2010. *Wisconsin executive summary: Allocation of scarce resources project.* Madison: Wisconsin Hospital Association, Inc. http://www.wha.org/scarceResources.aspx (accessed February 14, 2013).

Wolf, Y. I., A. Nikolskaya, J. L. Cherry, C. Viboud, E. Koonin, and D. J. Lipman. 2010. Projection of seasonal influenza severity from sequence and serological data. *PLoS Currents* 2:RRN1200.

3: Toolkit Part 1: Introduction

During a disaster, decision makers, health care providers, responders, and the general public are confronted with novel and urgent situations. Efficient, effective, and rapid operational decision-making approaches are required to help the emergency response system take proactive steps and use resources effectively to provide patients with the best possible care given the circumstances. It is also essential to develop fair, just, and equitable processes for making decisions during catastrophic disasters in which there are not enough resources to provide all patients with the usual level of care. Decision-making approaches should be designed to address a rapidly evolving, dynamic, and often chaotic set of circumstances. Information is often incomplete and contradictory. Agencies and stakeholders need to understand what information is available to support operational decision making in this kind of situation, and what triggers may automatically activate particular responses or may require expert analysis prior to a decision. This toolkit is intended to help agencies and stakeholders have these discussions.

TOOLKIT OBJECTIVE

The objective of this toolkit is to facilitate a series of meetings at multiple tiers (individual agency and organization, coalition, jurisdiction, region, and state) about indicators and triggers that aid decision making about the provision of care in disasters and public health and medical emergencies. Specifically, the toolkit focuses on indicators and triggers that guide transitions along the continuum of care, from *conventional* standards of care to *contingency* surge response and standards of care to *crisis* surge response and standards of care, and back toward *conventional* standards of care. The toolkit is intended as an instrument to drive planning and policy for disaster response, as well as to facilitate discussions among stakeholders that will help ensure coordination and resiliency during a response.

Box 3-1 presents descriptions of key terms and concepts. This toolkit (presented in Chapters 3-9 of the report) is designed to be able to stand alone, although interested readers will find additional background information and more nuanced discussion of key concepts related to indicators and triggers in Chapters 1 and 2.

This toolkit focuses on operational planning and the development of indicators and triggers for crisis standards of care (CSC). Public engagement is also a key element of CSC planning; a toolkit for community conversations on CSC is available in the Institute of Medicine's report *Crisis Standards of Care: A Systems Framework for Catastrophic Disaster Response* (IOM, 2012).

USING THE TOOLKIT

Toolkit Design

The discussion toolkit is structured around two scenarios (one slow-onset and one no-notice), a series of key questions for discussion, and a set of example tables. The example indicators and triggers encompass both clinical and administrative indicators and triggers. The toolkit is designed to facilitate discussion to drive the planning process.

Trigger: A decision point that is based on changes in the availability of resources that requires adaptations to health care services delivery along the care continuum (contingency, crisis, and return toward conventional).

Crisis care trigger: The point at which the scarcity of resources requires a transition from contingency care to crisis care, implemented within and across the emergency response system. This marks the transition point at which resource allocation strategies focus on the community rather than the individual.

Steps for Developing Useful Indicators and Triggers

The following four steps should be considered at the threshold from conventional to contingency care, from contingency to crisis care, and in the return to conventional care. They should also be considered for both slow-onset and no-notice incidents.

1. **Identify key response strategies and actions** that the agency or facility would use to respond to an incident. (Examples include disaster declaration, establishment of an emergency operations center [EOC] and multiagency coordination, establishment of alternate care sites, and surge capacity expansion.)
2. **Identify and examine potential indicators** that inform the decision to initiate these actions. (Indicators may be comprised of a wide range of data sources, including, for example, bed availability, a 911 call, or witnessing a tornado.)
3. **Determine trigger points** for taking these actions.
4. **Determine tactics** that could be implemented at these trigger points.

Note: Specific numeric **"bright line"** thresholds for indicators and triggers are concrete and attractive because they are easily recognized. For certain situations they are relatively easy to develop (e.g., a single case of anthrax). However, for many situations the community/agency actions are not as clear-cut or may require significant data analysis to determine the point at which a reasonable threshold may be established (e.g., multiple cases of diarrheal illness in a community). In these situations, it is important to define who is notified, who analyzes the information, and who can make the decision about when and how to act on it.

This chapter provides part 1 of the toolkit, which covers material that is relevant to all components of the emergency response system, including the scenarios and a set of overarching questions. Part 2 of the toolkit is provided in Chapters 4-9, which are each aimed at a key component of the emergency response system: emergency management, public health, behavioral health, emergency medical services (EMS), hospital and acute care, and out-of-hospital care. These chapters provide additional questions intended to help participants drill down on the key issues for their own discipline. These chapters also contain a table that provides example indicators, triggers, and tactics across the continuum of care. This is followed by a blank table for participants to complete.[1] The scenarios, questions, and example table are intended to help facilitate discussion around filling in the blank table.

These scenarios are provided to facilitate discussion and encourage practical thinking, but participants

---

[1] The blank table for participants to complete can be downloaded from the project's website: www.iom.edu/crisisstandards.

should consider a range of different scenarios—based on their Hazard Vulnerability Analysis—when developing indicators and triggers for their organization, jurisdiction, and/or region. The toolkit provides examples, but does not provide specific indicators and triggers for adoption. This discussion sets a foundation for future policy work, planning, and exercises related to CSC planning and disaster planning in general. The indicators and triggers developed for CSC planning purposes are subject to change over time as planned resources become more or less available or circumstances change. It will be important to regularly review and update CSC plans, including indicators and triggers.

Overarching Key Participants

This toolkit has been designed to be scalable for use at multiple levels. Discussions need to occur at the facility, organization, and agency levels to reflect the level of detail about organizational capabilities that is needed for operational decision making. Discussions also need to occur at higher levels of the emergency response system to ensure regional consistency and integration; it is important to understand the situation in other organizations and components of the emergency response system instead of moving unilaterally to a more limited level of care. Depending on the specific community, these discussions may be initiated at different tiers and may occur in a top-down or bottom-up fashion, but at some point, they must occur at all tiers reflected in the Medical Surge Capacity and Capability (MSCC) framework shown in Figure 3-1 (repeated here from Chapter 1). The development of indicators and triggers could be used by planners as an opportunity to benchmark their approaches, thus facilitating both intrastate and interstate coordination. This may be particularly valuable to entities operating in multistate locations.

This planning process is important regardless of the size of an agency; local preparedness is a key element of avoiding reaching CSC. Instead of using the MSCC framework and creating another response framework, some states may have existing regional and state infrastructures for inclusive trauma/EMS advisory councils/committees; the points made above about the importance of including all response partners and ensuring horizontal and vertical integration within and across tiers apply equally, regardless of the specific framework used.

The following participants should be considered for these discussions; additional participants may be brought in for the stakeholder-specific discussions and are listed in subsequent chapters:

- State and local public health agencies;
- State disaster medical advisory committee;
- State and local EMS agencies (public and private);
- State and local emergency management agencies;
- Health care coalitions (HCCs) and their representative health care organizations, and where appropriate, U.S. Department of Veterans Affairs Medical Centers and Military Treatment Facilities that are part of those HCCs;
- State associations, including hospital, long-term care, home health, palliative care/hospice, and those that would reach private practitioners;
- State and local law enforcement agencies;
- State and local elected officials;

- State and local behavioral health agencies;
- Legal representatives and ethicists; and
- Nongovernmental organizations that may be impacted by implementation of CSC (AABB, American Red Cross local chapter, etc.).

When Should These Discussions Take Place?

For communities that have already begun to develop CSC plans, this toolkit can be used to specifically develop the indicators and triggers component of the plan. For communities that are in the early phases of the CSC planning process, the use of this toolkit, and the exploration of community-, regional-, and state-derived indicators, triggers, and the process by which actions are then taken, would be an excellent place to start this important work. It provides much of the needed granularity about what it means to transition away from conventional response and toward the delivery of health care that occurs in the contingency arena, or in worst cases, under crisis conditions. For additional guidance on the development of CSC plans, including planning milestones and templates, see the Institute of Medicine's (IOM's) 2012 report.

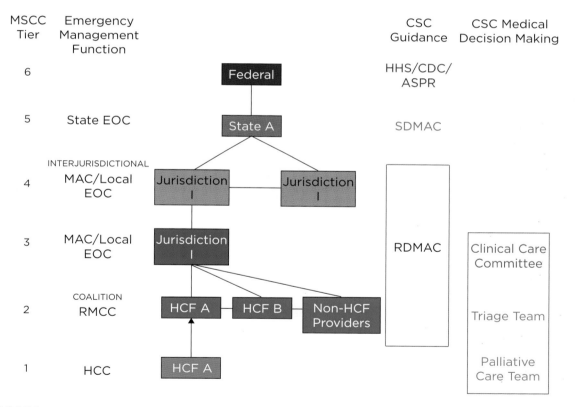

FIGURE 3-1
Integrating crisis standards of care planning into the Medical Surge Capacity and Capability framework.
NOTES: See Table 2-2 in IOM (2012) for further detail and description of the functions of these entities. The clinical care committee, triage team, and palliative care team may be established at MSCC tiers 1, 2, or 3. The RDMAC may be established at MSCC tiers 2, 3, or 4, depending on local agreements. The RMCC is linked to the MAC/Local EOC and is intended to provide regional health and medical information in those communities; it functions at MSCC tiers 2-4. ASPR = Assistant Secretary for Preparedness and Response (Department of Health and Human Services); CDC = Centers for Disease Control and Prevention; CSC = crisis standards of care; EOC = emergency operations center; HCC = health care coalition; HCF = health care facility; HHS = Department of Health and Human Services; MAC = Medical Advisory Committee; RDMAC = Regional Disaster Medical Advisory Committee; RMCC = Regional Medical Coordination Center; SDMAC = State Disaster Medical Advisory Committee.
SOURCE: Adapted from IOM, 2012, p. 1-44.

Suggested Process

As noted above, discussions should occur at multiple tiers of the system. A suggested process is provided in Figure 3-2 for discussions at the level of the health care organization, agency, or a small number of related agencies (e.g., EMS and dispatch).

For discussions at higher tiers of the system (e.g., among organizations, coalitions, and agencies from multiple sectors), additional work by participants in advance would be helpful so they arrive having already given thought to the indicators, triggers, and tactics that their own organization or agency would expect to use. Depending on whether this series of discussions is occurring top-down or bottom-up in a given community, this advance work could be done through convening sector-specific discussions first, as described above, or simply through asking each participant to start thinking about his or her own organization's or agency's likely actions beforehand.

In particular, it is important to highlight that the two government entities, emergency management and public health, should review the other sections and ensure that the activities they have outlined would support the activities described in the other sections. This would solidify the intent that local and state governmental agencies will need to support health care organizations and HCCs during CSC.

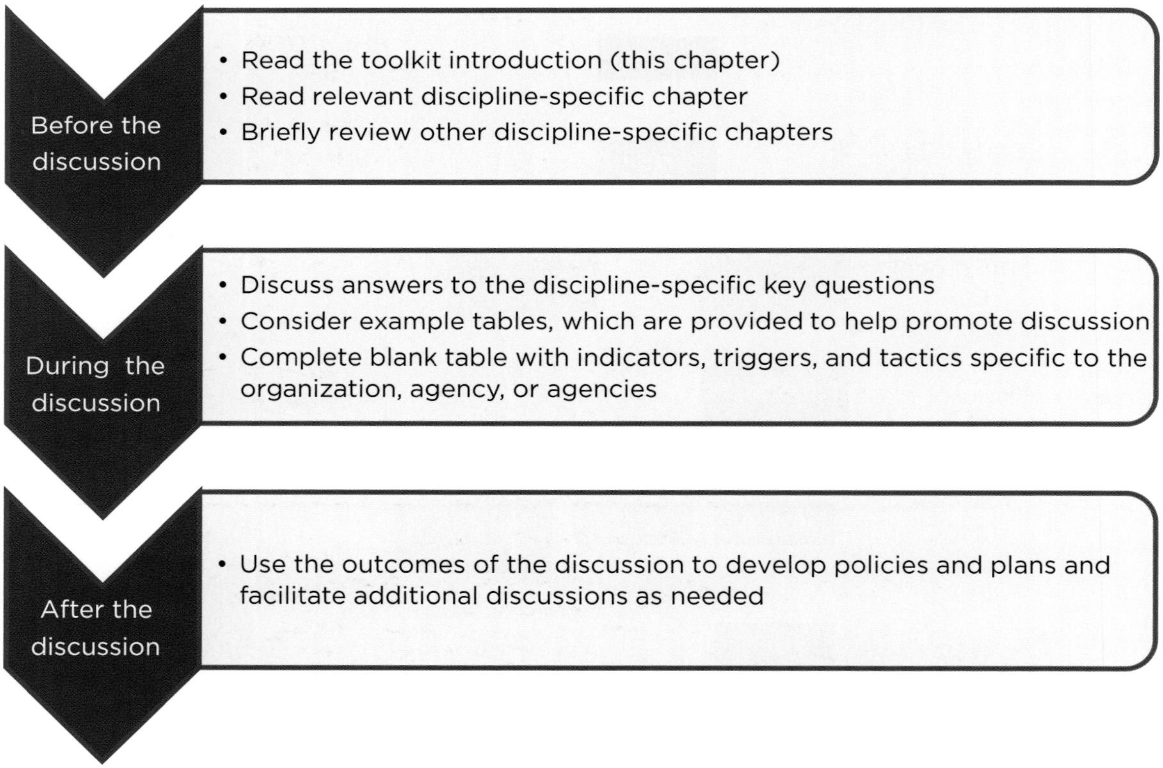

Before the discussion
- Read the toolkit introduction (this chapter)
- Read relevant discipline-specific chapter
- Briefly review other discipline-specific chapters

During the discussion
- Discuss answers to the discipline-specific key questions
- Consider example tables, which are provided to help promote discussion
- Complete blank table with indicators, triggers, and tactics specific to the organization, agency, or agencies

After the discussion
- Use the outcomes of the discussion to develop policies and plans and facilitate additional discussions as needed

FIGURE 3-2
Suggested discussion process.
NOTES: The example tables are provided to help facilitate discussion and provide a sense of the level of detail and concreteness that will be valuable; they are not intended to be exhaustive or universally applicable. It is important that participants complete the blank table with key indicators, triggers, and tactics that are specific to their organization, agency, or agencies. Depending on the size of the discussion group, it may be most useful for a subgroup of participants to develop the next steps.

To ensure that this aspect of CSC planning is not done in isolation, it would be helpful if the person(s) leading this initiative has/have more in-depth knowledge of the IOM's 2012 report, in addition to knowledge about the emergency preparedness program within their facility, agency, and/or jurisdiction.

Assumptions

This toolkit assumes that participants have an understanding of baseline resource availability and demand in their agency, jurisdiction, and/or region. The toolkit focuses on detecting movement away from that baseline, and associated decision making.

This toolkit presents common questions, ideas for discussion issues, and example indicators and triggers. Because the availability of resources varies across communities, it is clear that the answers will look very different. That is why this toolkit is a starting point for discussions and is not prescriptive.

Because communities across the nation are at different stages of planning, this toolkit could be used to fill a specific gap in an existing CSC plan, but it also could serve as a first entry point into a larger CSC planning effort.

SLOW-ONSET SCENARIO (PANDEMIC INFLUENZA)[2]

In early fall, a novel influenza virus was detected in the United States. The virus exhibited twice the usual expected influenza mortality rate. As the case numbers increased, a nationwide pandemic was declared. The Centers for Disease Control and Prevention (CDC) identified the at-risk populations as school-aged children, middle-aged asthmatics, all smokers, and individuals greater than age 62 with underlying pulmonary disease. Vaccine for the novel virus is months away.

Emergency Management

Emergency management has been in communication with public health as this outbreak has unfolded, maintaining situational awareness. They have initiated planning with all key stakeholders as soon as the pandemic was recognized. The county emergency operations center (EOC) was activated, first virtually, then partially, and then fully, as cases began to overwhelm the medical and public health systems. Emergency management has been responding to the logistical needs of public health, EMS, and the medical care system and is coordinating information through a Joint Information System. At the request of local EOCs and the State Health Emergency Coordination Center, the State Emergency Operation Center has been activated. The key areas of focus are coordinating volunteers, providing security, maintaining and augmenting communications, and facilitating coordination of efforts in support of the Emergency Support Function (ESF)-8 agencies. The emergency managers maintain the incident planning cycle and assist ESF-8 personnel in writing daily incident action plans and determining resource needs and sources. Private corporations have given significant support, lending personnel to staff points of dispensing sites, providing home meals to those isolated in their homes or on self-quarantine, and providing logistical support to hotlines and

---

[2] The two scenarios presented here have been adapted from the two scenarios in Appendix C of IOM (2009). They are provided to encourage discussion and practical thinking, but participants should not confine themselves to the specific details of the scenarios and should consider a range of scenarios based on their Hazard Vulnerability Analysis.

alternate care sites. Later on, when the pandemic winds down, the EOC will help coordinate transition of services toward conventional footing and identify the necessary resources to recovery planning and after-action activities.

Public Health

Local and state public health have been monitoring the status and planning for the pandemic since it was identified through epidemiological data. Multiple health alerts have been issued over the past weeks as conditions or predictions changed and recommendations for targeted use of antiviral medications have been communicated by the State Public Information Officer based on CDC recommendations. Public information campaigns begin, and emergency management and public health convene planning meetings involving key health and medical stakeholders in anticipation of a sustained response. As noted above, vaccine is months away and, when it arrives, may initially be available in only limited quantities. CDC is recommending use of N95 respirators for health care workers. There is an immediate shortfall of N95 respirators in supply chains nationwide and local shortages of antivirals are reported.

Enhanced influenza surveillance has become a standard across the United States and the world. Local health care organizations increased influenza testing and the state laboratory has confirmed that the current strain of influenza virus is present in multiple counties statewide. Volume of laboratory testing has increased substantially in local, regional, and statewide laboratories, which are now looking at current resources and possible modifications to testing protocols.

As the epidemic expands, local and state health EOCs are active 24/7 to support the response. The lead for this incident is the ESF-8, and communications between local and state EOCs in collaboration with the State Health Emergency Coordination Center have been augmented and standardized. Declarations of emergency have been released from the state, including public health emergencies or executive orders consistent with state authorities. Public health and state EMS offices are preparing specific regulatory, legal, and policy guidance in anticipation of the peak impact and subsequent waves. In addition to the activities associated with health, state, and local public health, offices are also addressing other functions, such as human services programs, water quality, food safety, and environmental impact.

EMS

Volumes of calls to 9-1-1 have escalated progressively over time, with high call volumes for individuals complaining of cough and fever. Many high-priority calls cannot be answered during peak hours due to volume. To divert non-emergency calls, hotlines have been established (where available) through which nurses and pharmacists can provide information and prescribe antiviral medications if necessary[3]; auto-answer systems have also been established to direct callers to Internet-based information.

The state EMS office has been contacted and necessary waivers are under way. The physician or physician board providing medical direction for the EMS agency and the EMS agency supervisor have implemented emergency medical dispatch call triage plans and have altered staffing and transport requirements to adjust to the demand. As public health clinics are overflowing with people demanding medical countermeasures (vaccines and antivirals), there have

---

[3] See Koonin and Hanfling (2013).

been several reports of violence against health care providers, thefts of N95 respirators from ambulances, and threats against EMS personnel by patients who were informed they do not meet the transport criteria in the disaster protocol.

A recent media report about the sudden death of a 7-year-old child of respiratory failure from a febrile illness has caused significant community concern, sharply escalated the demand on emergency medical dispatch and EMS, and increased workforce attrition throughout the entire emergency response and health care systems.

Hospital

Hospitals have activated their hospital incident command system and moved from conventional care to contingency care as the pandemic worsens. These modifications have been communicated through their regional health care coalition to their local EOC with anticipated support and possible waivers. As patient volumes escalate to nearly double the usual volume, elective surgeries are reduced, intensive care unit patients are boarded in step-down units, inpatients are boarded in procedure and postanesthesia care, and rapid screening and treatment areas are set up in areas apart from the emergency department (ED) for those who are mildly ill. As demand increases, hospital incident commanders are convening their clinical care committees to work with the planning section to prioritize available hospital resources to meet demand, as well as anticipating those resources that may soon be in short supply, including ventilators. Hospitals are sharing ED and inpatient data with the health department. Requests for new epidemiologic and other data have been received. Schools have been dismissed and this, in addition to provider illness, is having a dramatic impact on hospital staffing, as staff who are caregivers are reluctant to use on-site child-care.

Out-of-Hospital

Home care agencies note a significant increase in the acuity and volume of their patient referrals as hospitals attempt "surge discharge" and triage sicker patients within their home. Many home care workers are calling in sick and the agencies are using prioritization systems to determine which clients will be visited on what days. Durable medical equipment across the state providers are starting to identify shortages of home oxygen supplies and devices. Ambulatory care clinics had to clear schedules to accommodate the volume of acute illness. Despite media messages to stay home unless severely ill, many patients are calling their clinics for appointments and information; this is tying up clinic phone lines much of the time. Clinics are struggling to keep infectious and noninfectious patients separated in their facilities. As the epidemic worsened, alternate care facilities started opening to augment care for hospital overflow patients. Hospice patients are being referred to acute care facilities because they can no longer be cared for at home and many do not have their advance directives with them. As the pandemic wanes, many patients who deferred their usual or chronic care during the pandemic, will now present to clinics and EDs, continuing to stress the outpatient care sector.

Behavioral Health

The pandemic has had a tremendous psychological impact. Nearly everyone is exposed to death and illness, either personally or via the media. Houses of worship and other gathering places where people typically get services and support are closed and people are feeling more isolated. Management of decedents is becoming problematic. Hospital and civil morgues and funeral directors are overwhelmed. Coffins and funeral home supplies are in short supply and there is difficulty getting more. Families of the deceased are becoming increasingly agitated and assertive, demanding that hospitals, medical examiners/coroners, and health authorities take action. Demonstrations about vaccine delays are occurring at hospitals, clinics, and the local health department. Interstate commerce has been affected as restrictions on travel and transport become more pervasive. This is resulting in a noticeable decline in the availability of goods and services. Police are reporting instances of aggression, especially in grocery stores and at ATMs that have not been resupplied. The local and state Department of Social Services is reporting increased calls regarding substance abuse and domestic violence in homes where families have sheltered in place.

Those with preexisting behavioral health conditions are destabilized and require additional support, and many in the population exhibit features of new mental health problems, including anxiety and posttraumatic stress disorder. Existing psychiatric patients are also exhibiting increased symptoms as they are not able to obtain their medications. Police, health care workers, and community leaders are reporting substantially increased demand on detox services, and hospitals are discharging chemically dependent and psychiatric patients to make room for other types of patients, which is contributing to some of the problems.

Health care workers and public safety personnel are particularly hard hit by stress, especially those who are not prepared mentally for resource triage. Efforts are being made to "immunize" targeted populations with information on normal and abnormal stress responses, and additional screening and crisis support phone lines have been set up. Conventional outpatient crisis care and inpatient psychiatric care are overwhelmed, and faith-based, volunteer, and other support organizations have to take a much more active role supporting those in crisis in the community. That support is increasingly difficult as needs become more pervasive and severe, and face-to-face individual and group support becomes more difficult.

NO-NOTICE SCENARIO (EARTHQUAKE)

An earthquake, 7.2 in magnitude on the Richter scale, occurred at 10:45 a.m. in a metropolitan area. It also affected multiple surrounding counties that are heavily populated. Along with the initial shaking came liquefaction and devastating landslides. This major quake has shut down main highways and roads across the area to the south, disrupted cellular and landline phone service, and left most of the area without power. Several fires are burning out of control in the metropolitan area. As reports are being received, the estimate of injured people has risen to more than 8,000. Deaths resulting from the earthquake are unknown at this time, but they are estimated to be more than 1,000. Public safety agencies are conducting damage assessments and EMS agencies are mobilizing to address patient care needs. Hospitals and urgent/minor care facilities have been overwhelmed with injured victims. Two community hospitals and an assisted living center report extensive damage. Patients and residents are being relocated to alternate care centers; however, these options are unsuitable for those requiring a higher level of medical support due to lack of potable water and loss of electrical power at several facilities. Outpatient clinics and private medical practices are woefully understaffed or simply closed.

Emergency Management

State, county, and local EOCs have been activated. The governor has provided the media with an initial briefing. As outlined in the National Response Framework, they are attempting to coordinate with EOCs in non-

impacted areas and neighboring states, as well as the federal government, in order to mobilize resources to send into affected areas.

Local EOCs in the impacted area are trying to gain situational awareness through damage assessments, communication with stakeholders about utility failures, road access, injuries, and structural damage. EMS and public health have representatives at the EOCs (public health represents the health care sector for the jurisdiction, including liaison to the health care coalition, by prior agreement). Widespread impacts on hospitals will require that those facilities be evacuated, but EMS is taxed by incident-related demands and difficult road access.

Public Health

The state ESF-8 agency has mobilized resources from unaffected areas and is working with the state emergency management agency/state EOC to request assistance via Emergency Management Assistance Compact (EMAC) for vehicles and personnel. The governors of the surrounding states have dispatched medical and search and rescue teams. Public health authorities are inundated with the flow of information and requests for public health and medical assistance coming in to the ESF-8 desk at the local level. The State Health Emergency Coordination Center is fully activated to support the health and public health sectors. Public health authorities are working to initiate "patient tracking" capabilities, and have been asked to support activation of family reunification centers. Health care facilities needing evacuation are calling asking for assistance, including the mobilization of additional personnel resources (e.g., Medical Reserve Corps). Coordinated health and safety messages are providing information pertaining to boil water orders, personal safety measures around gas leaks, downed power lines and active fires, and a description of what resources are being mobilized to respond to this catastrophic disaster event.

EMS and First Responders

Uncontrolled fires have erupted due to broken gas lines. The local fire agencies are unable to respond to all requests for assistance due to broken water lines, difficult access, and the number of fires and damaged structures that have been reported. Only priority structure fires (e.g., fires in or near buildings suspected of containing occupants or hazardous materials) are receiving assistance. Fire departments from counties experiencing less damage are sending whatever assistance they can; however, they are not expected to arrive before evening. Dispatch centers are initiating mutual aid from unaffected counties within the state on request of local and county incident command (IC) through their respective EOCs.

The 9-1-1 emergency lines are inoperable as telephone service has been interrupted by widespread power outages and downed cell towers. The 700 and 800 MHz radios are the most reliable communication because landline and cellular telephone service are inoperative. Many of the injured cannot reach local hospitals due to damaged roads, debris, broken water lines, and power outages that have slowed traffic to a near stand-still. EMS providers report a shortage of staff and vehicles. Air ambulances are temporarily grounded due to foggy and windy conditions, and commercial airports have been closed for an unknown period of time. Unified command has been established and casualty collection points are being identified.

The main freeway is closed due to several collapsed overpasses and road damage, the worst of which has occurred at the freeway interchange. The travel lanes on the overpasses have completely collapsed, trapping at least 12 cars and 2 tourist buses below. The Department of Transportation is assessing structural damage on all freeway overpasses.

The collapse of this segment of the freeway has obstructed or delayed the ability of ambulances and emergency response units to respond to 9-1-1 calls or transport to the local tertiary care facility.

The governor has requested assistance from the Federal Emergency Management Agency (FEMA), including a Presidential Declaration of Disaster. FEMA will initiate a Joint Field Office as a first step to coordinating federal support for this area. State emergency management has requested EMAC assistance for vehicles and personnel. Governors of surrounding states have dispatched medical and search and rescue teams.

Hospital Care

At one of the hospitals, a 300-bed Level 2 trauma center is occupied at full census, but the administrator activates the Hospital Incident Command System, which opens the hospital command center and activates the disaster response plan. Other area hospitals are also impacted. A damage report reveals that this trauma center is on back-up power and the water supply is disrupted, but there is no major structural damage. Victims are already arriving in the parking lot on foot and by private vehicle as well as by EMS transport. The interhospital radio system is still active, with multiple hospitals reporting significant damage to their hospitals and surrounding routes of access. The administrator recognizes that despite their limitations, they will have to provide stabilizing care to arriving patients. There is no need to imminently evacuate the facility, though appeals for additional staff and a status report are made to the health care coalition coordinating hospitals via radio.

Additional surge care areas are established in the lobby area for ambulatory patients and in an ambulatory procedure area for nonambulatory patients. Surgeons perform basic "bailout" procedures, but the sterile supply department will have difficulty resterilizing surgical trays with available potable water. The administrator works with established material management departments and hospital staff to take stock of materials that may be in shortage and recommend conservation strategies for oxygen, medications (including antibiotics and tetanus vaccine), and other supplies. Off-shift staff members are having trouble accessing the hospital, and many staff present are not able to reach family members—some have left to go find their families, some have stayed to work extra shifts. Blood supply is limited, with resources already being used for the first cases to arrive. There are limited capabilities to manage burn patients, which are usually transferred to the regional burn center. Health care coalitions in the affected area, as well as neighboring regions, are activated to support response.

Out-of-Hospital Care

Ambulatory care clinics, private medical practices, skilled nursing and assisted living facilities, dialysis centers, and home health care services are all significantly impacted by the earthquake. Victims of the earthquake and those patients unaffected directly by the disaster, but in need of ongoing support for their chronic medical care services, are all impacted. Patients requiring regularly scheduled dialysis are unable to receive care at their normal dialysis site. Patients dependent on home ventilators are concerned that their back-up power resources, if any, are not likely to last for more than a few hours. The regional health care coalition hospital coordination center works with public health in the local EOC to identify resources for these patients, including the identification of "shelter" options, but many simply head to the hospital as a safe haven. Health care practitioners and professionals are urgently recruited to assist in the establishment of alternate care sites and shelter environments, which are being set up around the perimeter of the most severely affected areas. Access to medications at pharmacies is significantly impacted, sending more patients seeking assistance to already overtaxed hospitals.

Behavioral Health

The behavioral health unit at the impacted hospital or social work department crisis response staff deploys a small team to respond to patient and staff mental health needs as a standard component of the hospital's emergency response plan. The hospital lobby is teeming with people who appear shocked and confused. The hospital sets up an emergency triage and assessment unit for persons with minor injuries and those survivors looking for family members, and initiates behavioral health assessment and psychological first aid, targeting those who appear to be disoriented or distraught.

At the hospital, uninjured citizens begin to arrive in large numbers trying to find their loved ones. The hospital has an incomplete and ever-changing list of those being treated and are challenged in the early hours to provide definitive answers to inquiries. Citizens are becoming more anxious and angry. Hospital personnel are attempting to physically sort and separate family members with loved ones being treated in the hospital, searching families, and families of those in the hospital morgue. The number of deceased patients in the hospital morgue is increasing from deaths related to the incident. In addition, community morgue resources are taxed.

Several people (including children) have experienced severe burns, local capacity has been exceeded, and burn patients have been evacuated to burn centers in neighboring jurisdictions. Searching family members are becoming increasingly agitated and demanding when they are unable to learn the whereabouts of their loved ones and/or be reunited with them. Communications about individuals' locations are being forwarded to governmental support systems such as local and state EOCs, Joint Information Centers, and nongovernmental emergency response agencies.

Some hospital personnel are refusing to come to work until and unless they can be assured of their safety in the hospital as well as the proper care and safety of their children (who are no longer in school).

At the request of local EOCs, the state EOC activates six Medical Special Needs Shelters, which are staffed with behavioral health assessment and intervention teams, and activates behavioral health crisis response teams to assist first responders active in rescue-and-recovery and evacuation activities. Rumors develop that registered sexual offenders or other "risky persons" are among those residing in shelters.

An inpatient forensic psychiatric unit has been damaged and deemed unsafe. Following hospital response plans, arrangements are attempted to move patients to a comparable facility in another county/state. Difficulties are encountered in arranging appropriate transport and the receiving hospital reports very limited bed availability.

The chaos associated with the incident has increased the public's anxiety that people will die from their injuries while awaiting emergency transport. Risk/crisis communication talking points are disseminated to local officials and the media as to where behavioral health assistance is available.

OVERARCHING KEY QUESTIONS

The following questions reflect overarching common themes that apply to all stakeholder discussions. The discipline-specific portions of the toolkit (Chapters 4-9) include questions that are customized for these disciplines; the overarching questions are included here to facilitate shared understanding of the common issues under discussion by each discipline.

- What information is accessible?
- How would this information drive actions?
- What additional information *could* be accessed during an emergency and how would this drive actions?
- What actions would be taken? What other options exist?
- What actions would be taken when X happens, where X is a threshold that would signal a transition point in care (e.g., cannot transport all patients, run out of ventilators, cannot visit all the sickest home care patients).
- Do the identified indicators, triggers, and actions follow appropriate ethical principles for CSC? What legal issues should be considered?[4]

WORKER FUNCTIONAL CAPACITY

It is important to highlight understanding and attending to the sometimes unique needs of those whose roles include administration of and response to an extreme incident. If their health (including behavioral health) is adversely impacted in ways that impact role function, the entire response can become compromised and, in extreme cases, fail. Preparedness activities should include detailed planning that anticipates and addresses behavioral health consequences for both decision makers and responders. Preparedness activities should address strategies for monitoring the responder population, identifying potential sources of psychological distress, and available interventions, including those geared toward stress reduction and management as well as resilience promotion among these responders. During a response, proactive monitoring of the "temperature" of staff is needed by supervisory personnel, with reports back to the IC, and aggressive measures to maintain morale, manage fatigue, and manage home-related issues for staff.

Table 3-1 below outlines indicators, triggers, and tactics related to worker functional capacity and workforce behavioral health protection. It has the same format as the tables included in the discipline-specific chapters that follow this one. These chapters provide tables with examples of discipline-specific indicators, triggers, and tactics; this is not an exhaustive list. The examples are provided here because this is a crosscutting issue that should be addressed by all sectors to improve the quality of decisions and quantity of available staff. The discipline-specific chapters also discuss strategies to address worker shortages.

Given the focus of this toolkit on decision making, the examples in the table are focused primarily on behavioral health and human factors. It is important to recognize that other areas of workforce protection, such as physical health and safety (including fatigue management), are also critical and should be considered during disaster planning processes. A comparable discussion should take place about other health and medical elements of force protection. In addition, the examples provided here are general approaches to worker functional capacity; for more details on individual topic areas, see the discipline-specific chapter and, in particular, the behavioral health chapter (see Chapter 6).

---

[4] Ethical considerations are a foundational component that should underlie all crisis standards of care planning and implementation. The Institute of Medicine's 2009 and 2012 reports provide extensive discussion of ethical principles and considerations. Considerations of legal authority and environment are also a foundational component to CSC planning and implementation. Certain indicators and triggers related to legal issues are included in this toolkit in Chapters 4-9; for additional discussion, see the 2009 and 2012 reports.

REFERENCES

Hick, J. L., J. A. Barbera, and G. D. Kelen. 2009. Refining surge capacity: Conventional, contingency, and crisis capacity. *Disaster Medicine and Public Health Preparedness* 3(Suppl 2):S59-S67.

IOM (Institute of Medicine). 2009. *Guidance for establishing crisis standards of care for use in disaster situations: A letter report.* Washington, DC: The National Academies Press. http://www.nap.edu/catalog.php?record_id=12749.

IOM. 2012. *Crisis standards of care: A systems framework for catastrophic disaster response.* Washington, DC: The National Academies Press. http://www.nap.edu/catalog.php?record_id=13351.

Koonin, L. M., and D. Hanfling. 2013. Broadening access to medical care during a severe influenza pandemic: The CDC nurse triage line project. *Biosecurity and Bioterrorism: Biodefense Strategy, Practice, and Science* 11(1):75-80.

TABLE 3-1
Example Worker Functional Capacity Indicators, Triggers, and Tactics for Transitions Along the Continuum of Care

Indicator Category	Contingency	Crisis	Return Toward Conventional
Worker functional capacity	**Indicators:** • Employees routinely working more than 150% of usual shift duration • Patient/public complaints increase • Worker complaints about coworkers increase (attitude, decision making, etc.) • Workers begin to exhibit increased signs of stress (physiological, psychological, emotional, behavioral, social) (unit supervisors should be passing on reports to the command center) • Increased sick calls • Coworker perception of excessive fatigue or maladaptive behaviors (inability to make decisions, increased anger, etc.) • Increases in role conflict issues (relative priorities of home/family well-being and job function) reported by unit supervisors or implied by infrastructure damage, school closings, or communications systems failures • Workplace accidents increase • Workers express doubts/problems with their perceived safety or education/training for current tasks • Negative media coverage/public perception of facility/agency response **Triggers:** • Worker signs of stress or fatigue (physiological, psychological, emotional, behavioral, social) become commonplace • Productivity/function begins to decrease to the extent that supervisory personnel must intervene • X% increase in errors/incidents reported formally or informally to command center • Increases in role conflict (relative priorities of home/family well-being and job function) results in increased difficulty covering shifts/key roles	**Indicators:** • Productivity declines further • Errors/incidents increase rate and severity (patients/public are harmed and/or die as a result of errors) • Facility policies and actions cause negative public/media attention or compromised function of operations/relationships • Role conflict (relative priorities of home/family well-being and job function) increasingly problematic • Workplace accidents continue to increase • Workers decline to assume responsibilities they deem to be high risk **Crisis triggers:** • Productivity/function problems due to personnel issues cause service disruption • Role conflict (relative priorities of home/family well-being and job function) results reach a point where units are unable to maintain staffing, patients are transferred to other facilities, personnel refuse to come to work • Unable to give workers time off between shifts, at least equal to shift length • Workers are noted to be falling asleep on the job or exhibiting other unsafe behaviors **Tactics:** • Intensify stress management/resilience promotion training and activities (e.g., psychological first aid) • Continue regular and accurate surveillance of stress-related issues • Continue integration of various stakeholders in strategy development and implementation (e.g., direct care leadership, administration, HR, general counsel, EAP, etc.)	**Indicators:** • Workers begin to exhibit decreased signs of stress (physiological, psychological, emotional, behavioral, social) • Productivity/function begins to increase • Errors, incident reports, complaints decrease • Decreases in role conflict (relative priorities of home/family well-being and job function) • Workplace accidents decrease **Triggers:** • Productivity/function return to baseline • Errors/incident reports return to baseline • Shift schedules and responsibilities return toward baseline **Tactics:** • Stress management/resilience promotion training and activities (e.g., psychological first aid) become routine part of organizational practices • Evaluate, enhance, and continue regular and accurate surveillance of stress-related issues • Continue integration of various stakeholders in strategy development and implementation (e.g., direct care leadership, administration, HR, general counsel, EAP, etc.) with focus on rewarding staff, memorialization where appropriate, appreciation activities • Scale back or discontinue specialized consultation from content experts in workplace stress • Review, evaluate, and appropriately modify personnel policies and practices • Deactivate mutual aid and other supplemental human resources

Tactics:

- Implement stress management/resilience promotion training and activities (e.g., psychological first aid)
- Implement fatigue management policies
- Ensure adequate staffing ratios or provide additional personnel support for non-expert duties (lower levels of trained personnel, etc.)
- Ensure incident information flow to staff (situational awareness) is maintained, including operational briefings and opportunity for staff to provide input and comment
- Liaison/discussions with collective bargaining representatives to avoid conflicts arising from disaster-related staffing changes
- Provide support for the staff's family needs (access to phone lines to call home, providing basic shelter to family members, child care, pet care, etc.)
- Provide appropriate nutrition support, including expanded hours of services
- Restrict nonessential duties (meetings, etc.)
- Ensure regular and accurate surveillance of stress and fatigue-related issues by management/supervisory staff
- Ensure integration of various stakeholders in strategy development and implementation (e.g., clinical care leadership, administration, human resources [HR], legal counsel, employee assistance programs [EAPs], etc.)
- Initiate staff appreciation activities
- Explore specialized consultation from content experts in workplace stress in extreme situations
- Review personnel policies and practices to explore ways in which stress on workers may be reduced, including rotations through other areas of the facility or variable responsibilities
- Review and update plans for mutual aid or other means of supplementing human resources

- Explore specialized consultation from content experts in workplace stress in extreme situations
- Implement changes in personnel policies and practices
- Activate plans for mutual aid or other means of supplementing human resources, including use of support personnel for all noncritical tasks

91

4: Toolkit Part 2: Emergency Management

INTRODUCTION

This chapter presents a discussion and decision-support tool to facilitate the development of indicators and triggers that help guide emergency management decision making during a disaster. This tool focuses specifically on the role of emergency management in supporting the public health and medical sectors during an incident that impacts conventional levels of care (although a similar discussion process could be used to develop indicators and triggers to guide decision making for a broader range of emergency management responsibilities). Because integrated planning across the emergency response system is critical for a coordinated response, it is important to first read the introduction to the toolkit and materials relevant to the entire emergency response system in Chapter 3. Reviewing the toolkit chapters focused on other stakeholders also would be helpful.

Roles and Responsibilities

Emergency management serves as the lead incident coordinating entity and thus supports the public health and medical (Emergency Support Function-8, or ESF-8) sector during a major disaster or incident via

- Facilitation of incident management process (including planning and operational cycles) and development of jurisdictional incident action plans;
- Public information and risk communication coordination (Joint Information System)
- Situational awareness and maintenance of the Common Operating Picture (COP);
- Resource request, management, and delivery logistics;
- Transportation coordination or support;
- Communications support;
- Mass care and sheltering;
- Public works, including road access and utilities support, and incident-specific safety;
- Legal and regulatory mechanisms, including the ability to co-opt resources and space when required; and

- State emergency management working with state health (or public health, as applicable) for requests for federal public health and medical resources such as the Strategic National Stockpile, National Disaster Medical System, or declarations related to health emergencies.

Key Issues for Emergency Management

Emergency management provides a critical nexus on which a major public health and medical response depends for success. The specific relationship between the other ESFs and ESF-8 are described in the introductory text (Chapter 1) along with an expanded overview of emergency management's importance to public health and medical incident response. A brief summary is included here to facilitate discussion and consideration during stakeholder meetings.

Emergency management should play an active role in facilitating and maintaining multiagency coordination with local public health, hospitals, emergency medical services (EMS), and other health care organizations; otherwise, it is extremely likely that the response will be negatively impacted. Pre-event planning specific to the role emergency management will play and the responsibilities of public health, hospitals, health care coalitions, and EMS agencies in various scenarios is critical to successful response. Lead agency designation and who represents the interests of the key ESF-8 stakeholders at the jurisdictional emergency operations center (EOC) is also a key issue to address prior to an incident as well as to confirm during an incident, so that roles and responsibilities are clear. Emergency management will likely play a lead role in community infrastructure protection, logistical support, situational awareness and information gathering, and facilitation of public information and risk communication dissemination. Public health will have the lead role in community-based health interventions (with logistic support from emergency management), policy development, containment measures, health surety (food and water safety, etc.), and public message development. Ensuring that the emergency management/public health relationship is synergistic prior to an incident will enable each discipline to concentrate on their responsibilities, maximize their respective resources and talents, and avoid duplication. This should also avoid confusion and unrealistic assumptions about the powers and abilities of each agency. This can only occur through joint planning, exercising, and response, which can begin with the structured discussions outlined in this project.

For the purpose of this toolkit, local and state public health will take the lead with their health care organizations and health care coalitions on the implementation of crisis standards of care (CSC) when conditions require. In some states, the state EMS office may reside within the department of health and be included in the leadership role. Emergency management will have a critical supporting role. Additional discussion about roles and responsibilities in planning for and implementing CSC is available in the Institute of Medicine's (IOM's) 2012 report *Crisis Standards of Care: A Systems Framework for Catastrophic Disaster Response*. This report also includes planning and implementation templates that outline core functions and tasks.

DISCUSSION AND DECISION-SUPPORT TOOL

Building on the scenarios and overarching key questions presented in Chapter 3, this tool contains additional questions to help participants drill down on the key issues and details for emergency management. It also contains a chart that provides example emergency management indicators, triggers, and tactics, and a blank chart for participants to complete. The scenarios, questions, and example chart are intended to provoke discussion that will help participants fill in the blank chart for their own agency.[1] Participants may choose to complete a single, general blank chart, or one each for various scenarios from their jurisdictional Hazard Vulnerability Analysis.

Discussion Participants

Suggested participants and key stakeholders for a discussion focused on emergency management are listed below.

Key discussion stakeholders: [suggested agency/jurisdiction primary participants]

- Jurisdictional EMS entities (public and private), including key medical direction personnel for each discipline;
- Jurisdictional fire/rescue;
- Local public health;[2]
- Hospitals/health care coalition(s);
- Local government legal counsel/authority;
- Medical examiner/coroner;
- 911 answering point(s)/public safety answering points (PSAPs); and
- County commissioner/board.

Secondary-level discussion stakeholders: [plans require integration with these partners]

- State emergency management;
- State public health;
- State EMS authority;
- State hospital and other associations;
- Elected officials and executive officers;
- State's attorney office or state legal representative;
- Law enforcement and corrections;
- Funeral and mortuary services associations;
- Faith-based and community volunteer agencies;
- Representative(s) from utility service providers; and
- Community stakeholders involved with management of large planned events.

---

[1] The blank table for participants to complete can be downloaded from the project's website: www.iom.edu/crisisstandards.

[2] As discussed further in the public health toolkit (Chapter 5), in some states there are no local health departments, only a (centralized) state health department that acts as both state and local. Even in those states with both local and state health departments, the state health department needs to be involved in the discussions. As noted in the two previous IOM reports on crisis standards of care (CSC), the local health department will focus on local and regional issues related to CSC planning, while the state health department will help to coordinate the local/regional planning efforts to ensure intrastate coordination and consistency (IOM, 2009, 2012). The discussion participants and stakeholders listed here are provided as a suggestion; discussion organizers should develop a participant list that would be appropriate for the structures and organization of the particular jurisdiction.

Briefing-level participants: [plans require awareness-level knowledge by these entities]

- Major local media; and
- Representative(s) from all local chambers of commerce.

Key Questions: Slow-Onset Scenario

The questions below are focused on the slow-onset influenza pandemic scenario presented in Chapter 3:[3]

1. What ESF-8 system information can the EOC and/or emergency management access? Do these systems integrate into the state-level incident management system (WebEOC®, ETeam®, etc.)?

2. How are hospitals, public health, EMS, and the rest of the medical care sector (dialysis clinics, nursing homes, etc.) represented at the jurisdictional EOC? If they do not have an assigned "seat" in the EOC, who represents their interests, and how are coordination and two-way communications maintained?

3. Is there a clearly delineated process by which these ESF-8 stakeholders advance resource requests to the local or state EOC?

4. What is the process by which the EOC communicates back to ESF-8 stakeholders about potential resource shortages and other challenges in other organizations/sectors (security issues, travel restrictions, etc.) that will affect their ability to function?

5. What declarations or legal/regulatory relief can help support ESF-8 response strategies during a major disaster (e.g., suspension of ordinances requiring transport to hospital by EMS)? What agency (local, state, or federal) has the authority to waive such requirements? Based on what information and at what point is the decision made to pursue these declarations?

6. How is a COP maintained during a prolonged incident or event?

7. What process is in place to ensure that timely, accurate risk communication is available and disseminated to media outlets?

8. What information from ESF-8 systems or other sources would lead emergency management to begin rumor control and management during a health event, and how would this be handled? Are health public information officials integrated into Joint Information Systems?

9. What information is used to monitor whether resources (e.g., law enforcement) are becoming overtaxed? What adaptive strategies and/or personnel can be used? Are Memorandums of Understanding in place to gain additional resources?

10. When does emergency management reach out to ESF-8 stakeholders to determine needs during a purely health-related event? At what point are virtual versus physical coordination locations used?

11. Does the jurisdiction have an active health care coalition that coordinates the medical aspects of incident response, and how can emergency management maximize these coordination resources?

---

[3] These questions are provided to help start discussion; additional important questions may arise during the course of discussion. The questions are aimed at raising issues related to indicators and triggers, and are not comprehensive of all important questions related to disaster preparedness and response.

Key Questions: No-Notice Scenario

The questions below are focused on the no-notice earthquake scenario presented in Chapter 3:

1. During a multi-jurisdictional incident or event, how are requests for resources prioritized when there are not enough resources to meet current requests?
2. How is utility outage and restoration information made available to the EOC and then to ESF-8 stakeholders (e.g., hospitals and their respective health care coalitions)?
3. What alternate transportation capabilities might be available to assist with evacuation in affected hospitals or health care organizations, such as skilled nursing facilities? Based on what information and at what point would the decision be made to implement these capabilities? What assistance is provided to health care organizations regarding decisions to evacuate or shelter in place?
4. What contingency plans are in place for regional staging areas and "automatic" regional mutual aid responses for public safety and EMS agencies after a catastrophic incident? Based on what information and at what point would the decision be made to implement these? Are additional contacts necessary with the state EMS and trauma office specific to the EMS role in response, and what information should be obtained prior to contact?
5. What process is followed when the traditional or legally authorized personnel and decision makers are unavailable to issue declarations?
6. How is situational awareness maintained with surrounding jurisdictions when widespread utility failures are possible?
7. How does emergency management support its staff (duty hours, sleeping areas, nutrition, etc.), reduce unnecessary workload, and provide family and staff with physical safety and support so that staff can make key decisions without impediments?
8. Do local and state emergency management have identified shelters, including those to meet the medical special needs clients in their jurisdictions?

Decision-Support Tool: Example Table

The indicators, triggers, and tactics shown in Table 4-1 are examples to help promote discussion and provide a sense of the level of detail and concreteness that is needed to develop useful indicators and triggers for a specific organization/agency/jurisdiction; they are not intended to be exhaustive or universally applicable. Prompted by discussion of the key questions above, discussion participants should fill out a blank table, focusing on key system indicators and triggers that will drive actions in their own organizations, agencies, and jurisdictions. As a reminder, *indicators* are measures or predictors of changes in demand and/or resource availability; *triggers* are decision points (refer back to the toolkit introduction [Chapter 3] for key definitions and concepts).

The example triggers shown in the table mainly are ones in which a "bright line" distinguishes functionally different levels of care (conventional, contingency, crisis). Because of the nature of this type of trigger, the examples can be described more concretely and can be included in a bulleted list. It is important to recognize, however, that expert analysis of one or more indicators may also trigger implementation of key response plans, actions, and tactics. This may be particularly true in a slow-onset scenario. In all cases, but particularly in the absence of bright lines, decisions may need to be made to *anticipate* upcoming problems and the implementation of tactics and to *lean forward* by implementing certain tactics before reaching the bright line or when no such line exists. These decision points vary according to the situation and are based on analysis of multiple inputs, recommendations, and, in certain circumstances, previous experience. Discussions about these tables should cover *how* such decisions would be made, even if the specifics cannot be included in a bulleted list in advance.

TABLE 4-1
Example Emergency Management Indicators, Triggers, and Tactics for Transitions Along the Continuum of Care

Indicator Category	Contingency	Crisis	Return Toward Conventional
Surveillance data (Scenario 1: Slow-onset)	**Indicators:** • Health alert: Novel virus reported causing illness in United States • Community epidemic **Triggers:** • Calls for additional resources and mutual aid increase from multiple local • Multiple jurisdictional and/or state emergency operations centers (EOCs) have been activated **Tactics:** • Activate incident planning process and communicate with key stakeholders • Establish operational periods and communication expectations • Communicate situation report to local EOC • Begin developing Common Operating Picture (COP) process	**Indicators:** • Novel virus causing epidemic affecting United States, and projected impact greatly exceeds available resources • Declaration of a severe pandemic **Crisis triggers** • None specified (surveillance data are not triggers for crisis care) **Tactics:** • Provide logistical support for Emergency Support Function- (ESF-) 8 sector agencies • ESF-8 planning/response driven by surveillance data—e.g., dispensing site or alternate care site security, volunteer staffing, transportation • Determine the level of service the agency will be able to provide • Coordinate information and response posture to state EOC	**Indicators:** • Event has been stabilized by the facility and the impacted community • Resources are returning to adequate levels based against the needs • Stabilization or reduction in the number of activated jurisdictional and/or state EOCs to coordinate resources for the crisis **Triggers:** • None specified **Tactics:** • Create demobilization plan for operations and systems monitoring • Provide support for documentation of surveillance data, their use, and archiving
Surveillance data (Scenario 2: No-notice)	**Indicators:** • Media reports of incident • National Weather Service (NWS) watches/warnings • Hospitals on emergency medical services (EMS) diversion **Triggers:** • Media footage of earthquake impacting community **Tactics:** • Notify emergency management group • Coordinate with stakeholder agencies to gain COP • Determine need for declarations • Develop initial risk communication/ public messages and publicize	**Indicators:** • Media broadcasts of catastrophic event in progress **Crisis triggers:** • NWS forecasts Category 4 hurricane landfall in 96 hours (or crest of flood that will inundate city center) **Tactics:** • Issue evacuation/shelter orders • Determine likely impact • Support hospital evacuations with transportation resources • Risk communication to public about event impact • Ensure health care providers can pass barriers to reach hospital	**Indicators:** • NWS forecasts • Damage assessments • Flood crest receding **Triggers:** • Safe conditions exist in evacuated areas **Tactics:** • Establish plan to reopen areas to public • Work with public health to protect returning citizens; e.g., communicate needs for water treatment, risk for infections/injury from cleanup, etc.

continued

TABLE 4-1
Continued

Indicator Category	Contingency	Crisis	Return Toward Conventional
Communications and community infrastructure	**Indicators:** • Impact on community, including transportation and communications infrastructure • Utilities monitoring information (grid monitoring) **Triggers:** • Loss of telecommunications capabilities to EOC or widespread community outages • Widespread road damage and debris from tornado **Tactics:** • Use alternate communications strategies, such as mass media and text messages • Public works clears roads to damaged areas to facilitate EMS/fire access	**Indicators:** • Community-wide and likely prolonged impact on infrastructure affecting large number of homes, transportation, and communication • Loss of potable water **Crisis triggers:** • Long-term loss of electricity • EMS unable to evacuate hospital and extended care patients due to flood waters **Tactics:** • Request National Guard high-clearance vehicles for transportation • Mass care shelters open • Open alternate care sites and shelters for patients with medical and functional needs in conjunction with public health consultation	**Indicators:** • Restoration of services and transportation access **Triggers:** • Restored electrical service • Increased supplies of potable water • Decreasing sheltered population **Tactics:** • Scale back tactics or revert to conventional operations • Transfer remaining patients with medical and functional needs to skilled nursing or other facilities
Staff *(Refer also to the worker functional capacity table in Toolkit Part 1 [Table 3-1])*	**Indicators:** • Increasing staff absenteeism • School closures **Triggers:** • Community alternate care or vaccination sites required **Tactics:** • Provide appropriate protection for staff (and families where relevant) to maintain their health and safety • Staff rosters should be referenced and calls to off-duty staff made for potential activation • Mutual aid partners queried for additional staff if conditions persist or resources become increasingly scarce • Coordinate personnel needs with ESF-8 partners and determine best source (local, regional, state, federal) • Initiate just-in-time or cross-training educational programs and protocols for qualified or eligible personnel to fill staffing gaps	**Indicators:** • Increasing number of alternate care patients, dispensing sites **Crisis triggers:** • Insufficient staff available to provide usual health care • Insufficient staff for dispensing sites/alternate care sites • EMS staff at risk of violence on scene due to disaster triage protocols **Tactics:** • Staff assigned to nontraditional roles • Staff augmented from nontraditional sources • Volunteer processing/vetting center initiated • Law enforcement support for EMS responders • Logistic support for any personnel brought into area through Emergency Management Assistance Compact	**Indicators:** • Decreasing numbers of patients attending vaccination sites, alternate care sites **Triggers:** • Vaccination/alternate care needs can be met with more limited hours/sites/resources **Tactics:** • Close specific sites and restrict hours of operation • Augmented and contracted staff can be released • Reduce staff hours and plan threshold for site closures

Space/infrastructure

Indicators:
- Hospitals at capacity
- Community interventions planned (e.g., vaccination, home quarantine)
- Displacement of populations
- Morgue capacity exceeds usual space

Triggers:
- Shelter or space required for public health response

Tactics:
- Use emergency powers and mutual aid agreements to obtain appropriate space
- Provide transportation or communications support for individuals on home quarantine (assistance with meals, hotline)

Indicators:
- Hospitals over capacity
- EMS unable to answer volume of emergency calls

Crisis triggers:
- Mass fatality event overwhelms morgue contingency capacity
- Alternate care spaces required for hospital patients—no remaining room on hospital campus to provide care

Tactics:
- Emergency repurposing or rededication of public space for patient care (gym, convention center)
- Emergency resources brought in to address infrastructure needs and shortages
- Request the dispatch or activation of mobile hospitals from their agent/ agency of authority and provide any regulatory relief that they or traditional health care facilities may need
- Provide regulatory relief for EMS to allow them to reconfigure crews and not respond to all calls according to emergency plans

Indicators:
- Evacuated areas opening again
- Epidemic interventions winding down

Triggers:
- Space needs for patient care can be met at hospitals again

Tactics:
- Support transport of patients back to hospitals
- Facility space is returned to its pre-event purpose
- Rented or purchased emergency and auxiliary equipment is removed and taken out of service

Supplies

Indicators:
- Vendor reports problem with supply/ delivery
- Supply consumption/use rates unsustainable

Triggers:
- Medication/vaccine supply limited
- Consumption rates of personal protective equipment unsustainable
- Vendor shortages impact ability to provide normal resources
- Requests for refrigerated trucks to expand temporary storage of decedents

Tactics:
- Supply levels are checked and estimates are made as to how long the current inventory will last
- Additional orders are readied in case demand exceeds supply
- Alternate vendors contacted
- Determine alternate strategies—e.g., conservation, substitution, adaptation

Indicators:
- Shortage of equipment and supplies
- Transportation resources unavailable
- Continued requests for mass fatality resources as capacity is exceeded

Crisis triggers:
- Shortage of critical equipment and supplies

Tactics:
- Emergency powers considered to co-opt selected supplies
- Facilitate non-standard delivery (e.g., via boat, snowmobile, etc.) of materials
- Work with state emergency management and public health for identification and process to implement temporary internment

Indicators:
- Inventory needs become matched to inventory available
- Procurement and delivery systems have returned to pre-event status

Triggers:
- Supply needs can be met through usual channels/adequate supply available

Tactics:
- Return co-opted supplies
- Track return and invoicing of leased/ loaned supplies

Decision-Support Tool: Blank Table to Be Completed

Prompted by discussion of the key questions above, participants should fill out this blank table (or multiple tables for different scenarios) with key system indicators and triggers that will drive actions in their own organizations, agencies, and jurisdictions.[4]

Reminders:

- *Indicators* are measures or predictors of changes in demand and/or resource availability; *triggers* are decision points.
- The key questions were designed to facilitate discussion—customized for emergency management— about the following four steps to consider when developing indicators and triggers for a specific organization/agency/jurisdiction: (1) identify key response strategies and actions, (2) identify and examine potential indicators, (3) determine trigger points, (4) determine tactics.
- Discussions about triggers should include (a) triggers for which a "bright line" can be described, and (b) *how* expert decisions to implement tactics would be made using one or more indicators for which no bright line exists. Discussions should consider the benefits of *anticipating* the implementation of tactics, and of *leaning forward* to implement certain tactics in advance of a bright line or when no such line exists.
- The example table may be consulted to promote discussion and to provide a sense of the level of detail and concreteness that is needed to develop useful indicators and triggers for a specific organization/agency/jurisdiction.
- This table is intended to frame discussions and create awareness of information, policy sources, and issues at the agency level to share with other stakeholders. Areas of uncertainty should be noted and clarified with partners.
- Refer back to the toolkit introduction (Chapter 3) for key definitions and concepts.

---

[4] The blank table for participants to complete can be downloaded from the project's website: www.iom.edu/crisisstandards.

Scope and Event Type: _____

Indicator Category	Contingency	Crisis	Return Toward Conventional
Surveillance data	Indicators: Triggers: Tactics:	Indicators: Crisis triggers: Tactics:	Indicators: Triggers: Tactics:
Communications and community infrastructure	Indicators: Triggers: Tactics:	Indicators: Crisis triggers: Tactics:	Indicators: Triggers: Tactics:
Staff	Indicators: Triggers: Tactics:	Indicators: Crisis triggers: Tactics:	Indicators: Triggers: Tactics:
Space/infrastructure	Indicators: Triggers: Tactics:	Indicators: Crisis triggers: Tactics:	Indicators: Triggers: Tactics:
Supplies	Indicators: Triggers: Tactics:	Indicators: Crisis triggers: Tactics:	Indicators: Triggers: Tactics:
Other categories	Indicators: Triggers: Tactics:	Indicators: Crisis triggers: Tactics:	Indicators: Triggers: Tactics:

REFERENCES

IOM (Institute of Medicine). 2009. *Guidance for establishing crisis standards of care for use in disaster situations: A letter report.* Washington, DC: The National Academies Press. http://www.nap.edu/catalog.php?record_id=12749 (accessed April 3, 2013).

IOM. 2012. *Crisis standards of care: A systems framework for catastrophic disaster response.* Washington, DC: The National Academies Press. http://www.nap.edu/openbook.php?record_id=13351 (accessed April 3, 2013).

5: Toolkit Part 2: Public Health

INTRODUCTION

This chapter presents a discussion and decision-support tool to facilitate the development of indicators and triggers that help guide public health decision making during a disaster or public health or medical emergency. This tool focuses specifically on the role of public health in supporting the public health and medical sector across the spectrum, from prehospital care through end-of-life care. Because integrated planning across the emergency response system is critical for a coordinated response, it is important to first read the introduction to the toolkit and materials relevant to the entire emergency response system in Chapter 3. Reviewing the toolkit chapters focused on other stakeholders would also be useful.

Roles and Responsibilities

Public health is a complex system focused on the health of the population residing within their jurisdiction. Activities focus on protecting people from unsafe or harmful conditions while providing methods to promote optimum health and prevent disease. Public health can be established as a local government function, sometimes called "home ruled," in which the jurisdiction has the authority to set up their own governance and local ordinances. These cannot be counter to overall state authority. State public health has responsibility for the health of the population within the entire state, and may consist of locally run satellite state public health agencies. In either model, state public health has powers under the authority of the governor outlined in state statutes, which can be enacted in a public health, natural disaster, or catastrophic medical incident when usual mechanisms and powers are insufficient to meet the regulatory or response requirements of an incident.

Threats to human health are always present, whether caused by nature or humans. Without thorough preparation and coordinated planning between government and private-sector partners, communities and individuals will be unable to prevent, protect against, respond to, and mitigate incidents, and rapidly recover when an incident occurs. Public health and medical preparedness can only be achieved when component partners at the local, regional, and state/tribal level work in synergy through all-hazards preparedness. This becomes critical when resources are scarce. Local and state public health should lead the planning for crisis standards of care (CSC) and ensure both an implementation plan and incorporation into the culture of the health spectrum.

Additional discussion about public health roles and responsibilities in planning for and implementing CSC is available in the Institute of Medicine's (IOM's) 2012 report *Crisis Standards of Care: A Systems Framework for Catastrophic Disaster Response*. This report also includes planning and implementation templates that outline core functions and tasks.

DISCUSSION AND DECISION-SUPPORT TOOL

Suggested participants for a discussion focused on public health are listed below. Building on the scenarios and overarching key questions presented in Chapter 3, this tool contains additional questions to help participants drill down on the key issues and details for public health. It also contains two charts (one for slow-onset and one for no-notice) that provide example public health indicators, triggers, and tactics, and a blank chart for participants to complete. The scenarios, questions, and example chart are intended to provoke discussion that will help participants fill in the blank chart for their own situation.[1] Participants may choose to complete a single, general blank chart, or one each for various scenarios from their Hazard Vulnerability Analysis.

The questions below and associated table of sample indicators and triggers are broken out by the two scenarios because the role of public health will vary significantly based on the incident. Nearly all incidents or planned events will need public health and medical assistance and possible response. The first scenario demonstrates a slow-onset incident in which local and state public health would monitor the activity of influenza worldwide. This would provide an opportunity for planning and anticipating response activities. The second scenario demonstrates the issues associated with a no-notice event and describes potential points of consideration to respond and support response activities. In this scenario, there will be an immediate role of medical response, supported by public health, and intermediate- and long-term responsibilities for local and state public health offices.

Discussion Participants

From a public health perspective, any agency or organization that will be impacted in their service delivery by public health decisions should be discussion participants at some point in the deliberation process.[2]

Public health impacts all sectors and thus the need for integrated planning and long-term follow-up should be a key component in planning for and implementing CSC and will have a critical supporting role throughout an incident.

Local public health discussions should include their agency emergency management/preparedness coordinator, health officer, and medical director at a minimum. Agency subject matter experts (SMEs) should be engaged based on incident type, with consideration of potential clinical services impacted: communi-

---

[1] The blank table for participants to complete can be downloaded from the project's website: www.iom.edu/crisisstandards.

[2] As discussed above, the structure and organization of public health and health varies across states and localities. The discussion participants listed here are provided as a suggestion; discussion organizers should develop a participant list that would be appropriate for the structures and organization of the particular jurisdiction.

cable disease, epidemiology, environmental health, legal, and any departments that serve vulnerable populations potentially impacted. Other governmental entities, such as emergency management, behavioral health, county commissioners, coroner or medical examiner, and other key stakeholders, should also be included.

Local **external** discussion participants would include executive leadership of the impacted medical organizations, such as hospital chief executive officers (or chief medical officer and/or emergency department medical director or nurse manager), medical director or executive of emergency medical services (EMS) agency(s), Federally Qualified Health Centers, long-term care facilities, community mental health, dialysis center(s), home care, impacted primary care providers, funeral directors, etc., for SME input as the incident expands.

State public health entities involved may be a chief medical executive, state health officer, state epidemiologist, director of public health preparedness, an EMS and trauma system medical director or executive, a behavioral/mental health executive, health emergency management coordinator (EMC)[3] and Emergency Support Function- (ESF-) 8 leads/state health operation center chiefs, and a legal advisor, including attorney general, if appropriate.

State **external** discussion participants would be the State Disaster Medical Advisory Committee (SDMAC) or designee, impacted local health agencies, regional health care coalition leadership or similar group (e.g., state EMS/trauma advisory committees), executive leadership of impacted medical health organizations (e.g., hospital association, state medical society, behavioral/mental health, state pediatric association) and other stakeholders or SMEs based on incident or event.

Key Questions: Slow-Onset Scenario

The questions below are focused on the slow-onset influenza pandemic scenario presented in Chapter 3[4]:

1. What routine medical and public health surveillance systems are in place? Who or what agency submits the data, and who routinely monitors? Are these systems integrated to ensure multiple data feeds such as electronic communicable disease and laboratory results, influenza-like illness, sentinel physician reports, and pharmacy and over-the-counter medication sales, etc.? In reviewing these systems, are there thresholds already established that trigger actions or the need for further public health review?

2. Is an emergency department syndromic surveillance system in place? What are the components, thresholds, triggers, etc.? Is a protocol in place for further investigation once a threshold is identified? How would trending data indicate or contribute to the local/state potential impact on delivery of services and standards of care?

---

[3] A state health emergency management coordinator (EMC) serves as the liaison from state health to the state emergency operations center (EOC). In this role, the state health EMC or similar role would identify collaboration or resources needed through other state agencies. Depending on the state, the entity coordinating on public health and health may be referred to in different ways, including, for example, state (public) health emergency coordination center, department of (public) health operations center, or state (public) health operations center.

[4] These questions are provided to help start discussion; additional important questions may arise during the course of discussion. The questions are aimed at raising issues related to indicators and triggers, and are not comprehensive of all important questions related to disaster preparedness and response.

3. What information would be communicated to the local or state emergency management that would trigger an EOC activation for a public health/medical event? How do incidents that have ESF-8 as the lead agency impact operations in the EOC?

4. Has the local or state health department identified triggers to impact or restrict public gatherings to minimize exposures and thus decrease demand for medical resources?

5. Because this is a slow-onset incident, is there a local trigger for request of Strategic National Stockpile (SNS) medical materiel through the state-identified process?

6. What is needed to initiate points of dispensing (PODs)? How does the health department identify the sequence of POD placement and staff resources? Are the hospitals closed PODs and are there any anticipated variations in planning and response during CSC activities? Will there be separate POD(s) for first responders and their families, and will this include off-duty as well as on-duty workers?

7. How does the risk communication/public information officer modify messaging to address evolving conditions and coordinate messages with other agencies? When and by what mechanism does the state or an interjurisdictional information system become necessary?

8. What is the status of the public health workforce? Does the individual agency have plans in place to identify and meet essential public health functions while supporting medical care delivery during CSC? How does the agency Continuity of Operations Planning impact delivery of services, especially if clinical services are offered within the public health agency?

9. How is the impacted workforce and a need to solicit and use volunteer health care providers addressed? For example, volunteers may be accessed through the Emergency System for Advance Registration of Volunteer Health Professionals (ESAR-VHP), Medical Reserve Corps (MRC), etc.

10. What data or information are/is needed by public health executive leadership to consider a declaration or regulatory relief to facilitate contingency or crisis care within the medical health community? What lead time is needed to educate and communicate with senior policy leaders?

11. What activity would follow a declaration of emergency by the governor (health or general depending on legal environment of jurisdiction) or executive orders by the local or state public health authority? Does the local depend on the state to generate? What is needed for the agency?

12. State public health—what is the threshold for activation of the SDMAC or engagement of other SMEs? What communications need to occur internally with state government?

13. A slow-onset incident with high mortality rate will impact ESF-8 activities specific to fatality management. What resources are needed to assist the local coroner/medical examiner? Are there local or state plans for surge of decedents that may include surge storage, temporary interment, etc.?

Key Questions: No-Notice Scenario

The questions below are focused on the no-notice earthquake scenario presented in Chapter 3:

1. What is the status of infrastructure within the impacted area and has public health identified what is needed to support response? This will vary dramatically with available health care resources at the local level and the degree to which they are impacted.

2. Do any governmental regulations or rules need modification to facilitate incident response? If so, what information is needed and which agency serves as the lead to modify (e.g., state vs. federal regulations)? An example would be an "1135 waiver"[5] (state request approved federally), modifications to regulations on spacing between patient beds, cribs, dialysis chairs (state), staffing ratios, etc.

3. What are the applicable public health authorities, and if actions are needed how and when are these initiated and by whom? These are often outlined in a state public health code, licensing regulations, or applicable legislation.

4. What unique information should be collected by local and state public health and provided to local and state EOCs to support the spectrum of health care response? What is the most efficient method to collect the information, which may include the health care coalition medical coordination center? This could include bed availability, patient tracking strategies, and anticipated shortfalls of equipment or supplies, etc.

5. What support is needed for impacted person tracking and/or family reunification?

6. What critical health-related services to the community have been impacted? Are resources available outside the immediately impacted area?

7. Can any of the impacted services be assisted by local or state public health agencies, such as public health laboratories?

8. Is there a secondary environmental impact to the health of the public in the impacted area (presence of nuclear power plant and hazardous materials production or storage sites, including "SARA Title III" sites[6]) for which local and state public health should initiate assessment and mitigation strategies?

9. How quickly and by what means can the risk communication and public information officer implement communication strategies in circumstances when usual means of communication are compromised? What additional resources may be needed to facilitate messaging in these situations?

10. What is the status of the public health workforce? What essential functions should be maintained and what resources should be mobilized to support medical care during CSC? How is the impacted workforce identified and paid, or volunteer health care workforce solicited and used (ESAR-VHP, MRC, etc.)?

11. What other governmental agency resources are needed to support response (priority contract access, transportation, vulnerable children/population services, vaccines, laboratory, etc.)?

---

[5] Waiver or modification of requirements under section 1135 of the Social Security Act. See http://www.ssa.gov/OP_Home/ssact/title11/1135.htm (accessed May 31, 2013).

[6] The Superfund Amendments and Reauthorization Act (SARA) of 1986 created the Emergency Planning and Community Right-to-Know Act (known as "SARA Title III" or EPCRA), which is aimed at enhancing emergency planning and "community right-to-know" regarding hazardous and toxic chemicals. For additional information, see http://www.epa.gov/agriculture/lcra.html (accessed May 31, 2013).

Decision-Support Tool: Example Tables

The indicators, triggers, and tactics shown in Tables 5-1 and 5-2 are examples to help promote discussion and provide a sense of the level of detail and concreteness that is needed to develop useful indicators and triggers for a specific organization/agency/jurisdiction; they are not intended to be exhaustive or universally applicable. Prompted by discussion of the key questions above, discussion participants should fill out a blank table (or a table per scenario), focusing on key system indicators and triggers that will drive actions in their own organizations, agencies, and jurisdictions. As a reminder, *indicators* are measures or predictors of changes in demand and/or resource availability; *triggers* are decision points (refer back to the toolkit introduction [Chapter 3] for key definitions and concepts).

The example triggers shown in the tables mainly are ones in which a "bright line" distinguishes functionally different levels of care (conventional, contingency, crisis). Because of the nature of this type of trigger, they can be described more concretely and can be included in a bulleted list. It is important to recognize, however, that expert analysis of one or more indicators may also trigger implementation of key response plans, actions, and tactics. This may be particularly true in a slow-onset scenario. In all cases, but particularly in the absence of "bright lines," decisions may need to be made to *anticipate* upcoming problems and the implementation of tactics, and to *lean forward* by implementing certain tactics in advance of reaching the bright line or when no such line exists. These decision points vary according to the situation and are based on analysis of multiple inputs, recommendations, and, in certain circumstances, previous experience. Discussions about these tables should cover *how* such decisions would be made, even if the specifics cannot be included in a bulleted list in advance.

TABLE 5-1
Example Public Health Indicators, Triggers, and Tactics for Transitions Along the Continuum of Care in a Slow-Onset Scenario

Indicator Category	Contingency	Crisis	Return Toward Conventional
Surveillance data	**Indicators:** • Epidemiologic data identify significantly increased or novel activity • Epidemiologic data identify unusual population affected • Trends over time indicate escalation and/or significant impact **Triggers:** • Health care organizations unable to submit data due to impact of medical surge volumes **Tactics:** • Investigate indicators further with additional data, case finding, etc., to attain improved situational awareness • Work closely with health care coalition and medical health partners to target data collection to key elements only • Develop additional data elements based on incident and potential workload impact • Consider what is already collected electronically and modify to minimize health care organization stressors	**Indicators:** • Epidemiologic data indicate benchmarks and thresholds for critical resources and maximum critical care capacity will be exceeded • (Fatality) Communications from local medical examiner or coroner that morgue/storage capacity has been exceeded **Crisis Triggers:** • Epidemic curves continue to rise with unclear peak of cases • Surveillance has to be modified to highest priority or impact-only with minimal set of identifiers for future follow-up **Tactics:** • Event-specific data collection to provide common operating picture and potential treatment/outcome information • Surveillance data collection narrowed to only automated data streams related to incident • Governmental entities waive communicable disease reporting rules to only that which is directly related to the incident and key health issues	**Indicators:** • Epidemiologic data indicate sustained decrease in "new" incident-related reports • Electronic reporting mechanisms indicate return to normal reporting processes by health care organizations **Triggers:** • Event-specific data collection is no longer required **Tactics:** • Public health initiates "catch-up" work to capture health data from the prolonged incident; this is a critical role for public health for future incident response and demand forecasting
Community and communications infrastructure	**Indicators:** • Communications systems (Health Alert Network [HAN], telephone, etc.) disrupted within and external to jurisdiction **Triggers:** • Multiple requests for assistance from multiple agencies or jurisdictions • Interruption or contamination of water supply or utilities • Identified need to establish communication hotlines • Requests for specialized services and needs for broad public communications	**Indicators:** • Continued need to communicate with public about high risk, evolving situation • Water supply contamination **Crisis Triggers:** • Reports of disturbances at health care organizations or public shelters, etc. • Prolonged and widespread utilities (power, natural gas) outages **Tactics:** • Use all established resources to coordinate and communicate health messages	**Indicators:** • Decreased requests for messaging • Decreased activity on established hotlines **Triggers:** • Media and health care requests returning to "normal" **Tactics:** • Continue to provide appropriate levels of communication to the media, community, and impacted health care organizations

continued

111

TABLE 5-1
Continued

Indicator Category	Contingency	Crisis	Return Toward Conventional
Community and communications infrastructure (continued)	**Tactics:** • Work with established media and professional organizations to ensure consistent messaging • Implement statewide hotlines through established mechanisms such as poison control center, 211, etc. • Coordinate risk communication strategies with governmental public information officials	• Increase availability of coordinated communications for gaps identified • Focused review of communications strategies to identify gaps in targeted populations vulnerable or causing disturbances	
Staff **(Refer also to the worker functional capacity table in Toolkit Part 1 [Table 3-1])**	**Indicators:** • Increasing absenteeism among public health staff; increased demand for staffing for community-based interventions, etc. **Triggers:** • Community-based interventions required (e.g., vaccine, countermeasure distribution, "flu centers") **Tactics:** • Eliminate routine or non-life safety laboratory testing, surveillance of community organizations, etc. • Initiate Continuity of Operations Planning to ensure that essential functions for local and state public health are implemented to support health care organization response • Identify services to put on "pause" as personnel resources continue to decline • Activate mutual aid/support plans from other agencies, disciplines, predesignated volunteer sources as required • Off-load tasks onto technology as possible (e.g., hotlines rather than face-to-face assessments) • Change staffing patterns and hours	**Indicators:** • Increasing absenteeism and inability to fulfill critical missions to community • Increased demand for resources **Crisis Triggers:** • Unable to fulfill critical missions (e.g., support alternate care sites) with appropriate staff **Tactics:** • Eliminate all nonessential functions to support local and state response to the incident • Reallocate any health professionals whose training allows them a more active role to support health care organizations • Assist if needed in coordination of health volunteers to support public health and medical functions identified • Triage personnel resources to services of most benefit (community vaccination, etc.) • Use just-in-time recruiting and training as required to fulfill missions • Obtain regulatory relief as required to facilitate facility crisis responses (e.g., who may administer vaccinations)	**Indicators:** • Impact of incident decreasing • Personnel absenteeism is decreasing • Personnel communicating need to initiate activities to "return to normal operations" **Triggers:** • Missions able to be completed with adequate staffing **Tactics:** • Review and prioritize key services for reimplementation at the local and state levels • Initiate data analysis of impact of crisis standards of care (CSC) implementation on personnel • Revert to normal staffing patterns/hours/duties

Space/infrastructure

continued

Indicators:

- Health care organizations are unable to meet demands with traditional bed capacity with all surge strategies implemented
- Local and state public health initiated strategies to authorize alternate care site initiation; this includes assurances related to governmental waivers

Triggers:

- Space expansion is required for community-based interventions (vaccination campaign, etc.)
- Recognition of the need to open alternate care sites for screening clinics/early treatment

Tactics:

- Requests are made for waivers to authorize alternate care sites for care delivery
- Local public health departments work with their local health care organizations and regional health care coalitions to ensure that inpatient sites, including skilled nursing facilities, are prioritized for support
- Public health provides risk communication and coordination assistance for medical care system—when to seek care, etc.
- Local health departments work with their primary care providers to identify mechanisms to expand services and protect personnel
- Emergency Support Function-8 lead to keep each local emergency operations center aware of impact and contingency care implemented
- State health implement statewide plans for nurse triage lines, 211, poison control support for callers related to event
- State public health works with all health care coalitions to support implementation of statewide medical surge strategies
- State health emergency coordination center to keep each local health department aware of impact and contingency care implemented

Indicators:

- Health care organizations have narrowed admission criteria to maximize available resources

Crisis Triggers:

- Health care organizations have implemented all medical surge strategies and should seek alternate care site locations for inpatient care overflow

Tactics:

- Supply or support mobilization of deployment of volunteer health professionals
- Implementation of governmental waivers to establish alternate care sites
- State emergency operation centers and health emergency coordination centers work with state and federal agencies to establish declarations and emergency order rules specific to the necessary tactics to respond to the incident
- State public health to communicate with state disaster medical advisory committee to review status of CSC guidelines and distribute to impacted health care organizations

Indicators:

- Surveillance indicates declining new infections
- Health care organizations are able to broaden admission based on available resources

Triggers:

- Decreasing census in alternate care sites within jurisdiction
- State observes multiple health care coalitions readying for demobilization of alternate care sites

Tactics:

- Support health care alternate care site demobilization strategies
- Patient records, resources, and supplies should be accounted for and returned as required; local and state public health departments mobilize resources to assist as available
- State public health works with local partners and nongovernmental organizations to communicate plans to return to conventional care

TABLE 5-1
Continued

Indicator Category	Contingency	Crisis	Return Toward Conventional
Space/Infrastructure (continued)	• State health to initiate process for implementing executive orders for public health emergency; may or may not implement at this time • Local and state public health begin planning strategies for CSC if anticipated event expansion		
Supplies	**Indicators:** • Local and state monitoring of supplies and inventory data indicate shortage/potential shortage • Benchmark supply availability to disease reporting and mortality data • Anticipate challenges with medical supply chain based on expanding incident; review communications from each health care coalition for the impact to their health care organizations **Triggers:** • Decreased availability of critical medical resources anticipated • Requests to health care coalition medical coordination center for allocation of regional cache supplies **Tactics:** • Prioritize resource allocation by urgency of need and risk • Determine time frame and availability from other vendors/sources • Review and update risk communication strategies specific to users of critical resources and community • State health emergency coordination center work with each health care coalition to allocate regional cache contents and other resources • State health emergency coordination center initiates internal mechanisms to move anticipated Strategic National Stockpile (SNS) materiel requests to the state emergency operations center	**Indicators:** • Demand forecasting/projections exceed available critical resources • No national source of specific supplies available **Crisis Triggers:** • Shortages of critical equipment, drugs, or vaccine present significant risk to persons who cannot receive them • National guidance on rationing distributed **Tactics:** • Focus allocation of scarce resources to maintaining critical social/public safety function (civil order maintenance) • Coordinated risk communication strategies are critical • Use government purchasing powers to support critical medical supplies • Maintain communications with federal SNS program • State and regional disaster medical advisory committees review triage guidance available and propose recommendations • State public health circulates guidelines on allocation of resources • Legal, regulatory, and emergency powers invoked as required to facilitate fair, planned allocation process	**Indicators:** • Vaccine manufacturers have increased supply chain so targeted groups for vaccination is expanded based on disease trends and ethical guidelines • Additional resources are obtained • Demand for resources (e.g., ventilators) is declining as event wanes **Triggers:** • Critical medical supplies are sufficient to meet the needs of the patients requiring them **Tactics:** • Continued, coordinated risk communication • Assessment if transition is temporary or likely to be permanent • Local public health should augment Points of Dispensing plans to meet demands when vaccination is expanded as vaccine is available • Demobilization of SNS • State public health to review CSC guidelines for possible revision based on resource availability

Fatality management

Indicators:
- Rising death toll
- Rate of deaths projected to exceed local capabilities

Triggers:
- Health care organizations are reporting an inability to manage the number of decedents within facilities
- Local medical examiners/coroners are unable to meet the demands of their jurisdiction with usual processing

Tactics:
- Local public health works with medical examiners/coroners to determine if the bottleneck is processing (medical examiner caseload) or body management
- Local public health contacts funeral home, mortuaries, morgues, or crematoriums to assess current impact on capacity and expansion capacity
- Local governmental agencies should identify potential cultural barriers to modifications in death processes and prepare strategies to address these
- Initiate strategies to expedite the completion of death certificates/investigations
- State public health investigates modifications to laws, regulations, etc., for dealing with decedents
- Governmental authorities initiate planning for possible alternate storage strategies
- Consider federal or state disaster mortuary team resources
- Consider temporary storage facilities implementation plan

Indicators:
- Funeral homes communicating limited resources to conduct funeral services
- Rate of deaths projected to exceed regional/surge capabilities

Crisis Triggers:
- With disaster plans implemented, fatality processing demand exceeds available resources and threat of civil unrest or decomposition is real

Tactics:
- Risk communication strategies coordinated at local and state levels
- Activation of all available mortuary resources, including response teams and expanded cremation and processing operations
- Governor declaration for expedited burials and/or temporary interment upon state public health recommendation. (NOTE: Requires extensive planning with multiple state agencies to identify a location, tracking, and personnel support to implement such a response to manage mass fatality incident.)
- Consider transfer of decedents to other locations for processing if required

Indicators:
- Number of deaths from influenza are stabilizing or sustained decline

Triggers:
- Decedent processing is able to be accommodated within surge or conventional systems

Tactics:
- Risk communication on decedent management
- Local and state public health, in conjunction with medical examiners/coroners, resume normal processes, which include funerals and traditional burials
- Alterations that had occurred should be addressed to return to "normal state," recognizing the complexity associated with variation in cultural and societal death routines

continued

TABLE 5-1
Continued

Indicator Category	Contingency	Crisis	Return Toward Conventional
Congregate gatherings	**Indicators:** • Epidemiologic models indicate person-to-person spread is prevalent • Multiple jurisdictions reporting that large gatherings implicated in outbreak investigations • Outbreaks linked to funeral services **Triggers:** • Epidemiologic data indicate increasing outbreaks directly related to known congregate gatherings in more than one jurisdiction **Tactics:** • Local and state review immediate and future large-scale venues for anticipated cancellation • Local and state recommendations on school closures • State public health readies quarantine guidelines working with governor's office	**Indicators:** • Statewide indication of high transmission in gathering settings **Crisis Triggers:** • Forced quarantine is required to prevent spread of dangerous pathogen • Public gatherings prohibited **Tactics:** • Executive order or governor's declaration to eliminate congregate gatherings • Quarantine orders implemented as indicated • Governmental agencies collaborate to enforce congregate-gathering bans	**Indicators:** • Decrease in evidence for person-to-person trends • Criteria for identifying "superspreaders" as individuals allows targeted interventions **Triggers:** • Sustained decrease in disease transmission trends **Tactics:** • Governor rescinds gathering orders • Initiate public gatherings • Local and state continue close monitoring of epidemiologic data to ensure continued decline and are prepared to reinstate bans if cases increase

TABLE 5-2
Example Public Health Indicators, Triggers, and Tactics for Transitions Along the Continuum of Care in a No-Notice (Earthquake) Scenario

Indicator Category	Contingency	Crisis	Return Toward Conventional
Surveillance data	**Indicators:** • Collection of Essential Elements of Information indicates disruption of services that impact local public health and health care organizations within jurisdiction • Local health department identifies specific population health surveillance data impacted by incident • Impacted persons are being taken to multiple health care organizations through traditional and nontraditional methods • Forecast temperature extremes **Triggers:** • Communications from health care organizations to their health care coalitions that many facilities have infrastructure damage • Communications from local emergency operations centers (EOCs) to state EOC (SEOC) that medical and public health have significant impact to service delivery • Incident disrupts medical supply chain; anticipate shortages • Unable to locate or track all patients impacted by incident **Tactics:** • Data collection to local EOC • State health emergency coordination center queries all health care coalitions to identify statewide impact to service delivery and plan response strategies (patient and resource movement) • Local health department implements focused assessments and modification specific to impact of incident for jurisdictional population • Implement patient tracking system statewide	**Indicators:** • Scope of incident indicates need to focus surveillance on key elements to support medical and public health operations • Communications indicate emergency management and/or American Red Cross or other nongovernmental organization establishing multiple sheltering operations • Incident-related injuries necessitate modification of surveillance strategies • Shelters established, need for augmented surveillance to protect shelter population **Crisis Triggers:** • Health care organization capacity is overwhelmed based on casualty counts and impact on health care infrastructure **Tactics:** • Collection of key information only to maximize/distribute resources or reunite families • Continue established patient tracking system and allow access by non-governmental and other organizations as required to facilitate reunification	**Indicators:** • Focused surveillance indicates diminishing impact of incident **Triggers:** • No additional victims being entered into system • Decreasing numbers in shelters and consolidation of sheltering services **Tactics:** • Return to routine surveillance activities • Extensive review of incident-specific surveillance data to determine long-term follow-up or further focused surveillance • Archiving of patient tracking from event

continued

TABLE 5-2
Continued

Indicator Category	Contingency	Crisis	Return Toward Conventional
Community and communications infrastructure	**Indicators:** • Initial and subsequent damage reports indicate substantial loss of 911 or other communications • Initial and subsequent damage reports indicate substantial loss of health care or residential infrastructure • Numbers of persons are missing and the pressure families are putting on 911 and other systems to find them • Disruption of roads impact ability to meet the needs of patient movement **Triggers:** • Requests from multiple health care organizations and health care coalitions for governmental assistance due to infrastructure damage • Significant reports of safety issues that could impact community, thus indicating a need for coordinated risk communication strategies • Local EOCs getting queries from health care organizations about utility restoration **Tactics:** • Support requests from health care organizations through health care coalition • Prioritize key public health activities to support critical jurisdictional needs and health care organization service delivery • Local public information officials work with media on health-related risk communication strategies • State public information officials working with other state agency and local public information officials for coordinated risk communications • Local EOCs establishing mechanisms to implement family reunification systems	**Indicators:** • Local EOCs and state emergency operation center are fully activated statewide to respond to catastrophic incident • Widespread loss of utilities • Widespread loss of critical communications (cellular, Internet, public safety radio, etc.) **Crisis triggers:** • Incident unfolding with health care coalitions communicating more than X% of facilities with significant infrastructure damage (the level of care provided by health care organizations and their roles in the community will impact the number of damaged facilities that cause a transition to crisis response) • Inability for multiple hospitals to remain in their current building without significant support • Multiple health care facilities require evacuation and inadequate transport resources to accomplish this • Local emergency management indicates a need to establish multiple shelters, including functional needs **Tactics:** • Continued need for risk communications to community • Identify needs of health care organizations in collaboration with health care coalitions • Local health departments should identify staff, including volunteers, to assist with public health issues in shelters, including those targeted to functional needs • State public information officials working with other state agency and local public information officials for coordinated risk communications • State working with locals to ensure that family reunification systems can meet demands	**Indicators:** • Public safety communications back online • Repairs to health care organizations provide the ability to repopulate or resume previous level of service **Triggers:** • Emergency communications systems reestablished **Tactics:** • Communicate deescalation of incident to community through established methods and using risk communication strategies • Local and state public health assist with assessments or surveys to clear impacted health care organizations for repopulation or resume suspended services

Staff

Indicators:
- Personnel availability impacted by access, family obligations, injury/direct effects

Triggers:
- Request for additional medical or public health personnel to support operations

Tactics:
- Identify cross-trained personnel to support services linked to incident
- Modifications to services will be based on staff available
- Plan to support response with volunteer health professionals (Emergency System for Advance Registration of Volunteer Health Professionals [ESAR-VHP], Medical Reserve Corps [MRC], coalition, etc.)

Indicators:
- Personnel availability impacted widely by access, family obligations, injury/direct effects
- Local infrastructure damage will prevent mutual aid in a timely manner
- Alternate care sites and shelters initiated

Crisis triggers:
- Multiple organizations requesting medical staff support and inadequate availability of staff via usual programs (ESAR-VHP, etc.)
- Specialty consultation unavailable to hospitals boarding burn, pediatric, or other patients due to demands or communication issues at referral centers

Tactics:
- Use available staff and provide support for nonspecialized tasks to maximize response
- Limit services to those related to life/safety issues only
- Facilitate out-of-area specialty consultation as applicable
- Use volunteer health professional if available
- State to seek additional personnel resources through federal programs (Department of Health and Human Services, Department of Defense, etc.)

Indicators:
- Decreasing use of alternate care sites
- Decreasing requests for staff support

Triggers:
- Health care organizations releasing volunteer and other supplemental staff
- Alternate care sites demobilizing

Tactics:
- Initiate processes to return staff to routine positions
- Implement demobilization strategies if volunteers were used

continued

TABLE 5-2
Continued

Indicator Category	Contingency	Crisis	Return Toward Conventional
Space/infrastructure	**Indicators:** • Emergency management has initiated shelters • Emergency medical services (EMS) reporting evacuations of long-term care (LTC) and similar facilities • Hospital data indicate capacity exceeded at multiple facilities despite surge capacity plan activation **Triggers:** • Local requests for assistance with patient movement • Inadequate EMS resources to accommodate demands **Tactics:** • Need anticipated to modify EMS transport protocols statewide and suspend specific staffing and other response requirements • Local EOCs work with regional health care coalitions to identify and prioritize transport resources • State health emergency coordination center to work on statewide available resources through health care coalition structure • State public health and SEOC identify additional resources through Mutual Aid Agreements (MAAs) or Emergency Management Assistance Compact (EMAC)	**Indicators:** • Communications indicate demand exceeds patient transport supply • Hospitals have inadequate space for victims **Crisis triggers:** • Requests to modify EMS transport protocols • Requests for alternate care sites for inpatient overflow **Tactics:** • State ESF-8 works to implement protocol waivers to support modified transport plans • State public information official communicates efforts to all medical health entities • State coordination of field hospital and patient transportation assets from state, EMAC, and federal sources	**Indicators:** • EMS indicates return to normal dispatch and transport protocols • Alternate care sites no longer required/use diminishing **Triggers:** • System data indicate returning to baseline transport status **Tactics:** • Support efforts to return EMS to normal operations and regulations • Support demobilization of alternate care sites and shelter medical support • Local and state public health staff gather all after-action reports, meet with key stakeholders to identify challenges, and plan to support future operations

Supplies

Indicators:
- Interruption in supply chain impacts resource availability
- Local use of resources exceeds supply (e.g., blood products, surgical supplies)

Triggers:
- Resource shortages reported, including medical material and pharmaceuticals
- Local request for Strategic National Stockpile (SNS) or cache materiel

Tactics:
- Local health care organizations work with their health care coalition to distribute regional resources, including obtaining resources from health care coalitions that are not impacted by the incident
- State Emergency Support Function- (ESF-) 8 should identify possible waivers, including the reuse of equipment and supplies within health care organizations
- Initiate process to request SNS or other materiel through state EOC

Indicators:
- Critical medical supplies are unavailable

Crisis triggers:
- Unable to locate additional medical supplies to support medical care, presenting a life/safety risk

Tactics:
- Local and state public health should continue to identify resources to support organizational response; this would include implementing MAA and EMAC requests for services and supplies needed to deliver care
- Executive orders or public health/ emergency declaration if needed to support altering the use of equipment, supplies, or human resources
- Public health guidance on allocation of specific scarce resources may be required, with input from state disaster medical advisory committee

Indicators:
- Mobilization of equipment, supplies, and resources to meet demand

Triggers:
- Decreasing requests for additional supplies to support response

Tactics:
- Data collection and financial accountability to assess impact of incident and plan for remediation of gaps
- Continue situational monitoring —is this a temporary or sustained improvement?

Decision-Support Tool: Blank Table to Be Completed

Prompted by discussion of the key questions above, participants should fill out this blank table (or multiple tables for different scenarios) with key system indicators and triggers that will drive actions in their own organizations, agencies, and jurisdictions.[7]

Reminders:

- *Indicators* are measures or predictors of changes in demand and/or resource availability; *triggers* are decision points.
- The key questions were designed to facilitate discussion—customized for public health—about the following four steps to consider when developing indicators and triggers for a specific organization/agency/jurisdiction: (1) identify key response strategies and actions, (2) identify and examine potential indicators, (3) determine trigger points, (4) determine tactics.
- Discussions about triggers should include (a) triggers for which a "bright line" can be described, and (b) *how* expert decisions to implement tactics would be made using one or more indicators for which no bright line exists. Discussions should consider the benefits of *anticipating* the implementation of tactics, and of *leaning forward* to implement certain tactics in advance of a bright line or when no such line exists.
- The example table may be consulted to promote discussion and to provide a sense of the level of detail and concreteness that is needed to develop useful indicators and triggers for a specific organization/agency/jurisdiction.
- This table is intended to frame discussions and create awareness of information, policy sources, and issues at the agency level to share with other stakeholders. Areas of uncertainty should be noted and clarified with partners.
- Refer back to the toolkit introduction (Chapter 3) for key definitions and concepts.

---

[7] The blank table for participants to complete can be downloaded from the project's website: www.iom.edu/crisisstandards.

Scope and Event Type: _____

Indicator Category	Contingency	Crisis	Return Toward Conventional
Surveillance data	Indicators: Triggers: Tactics:	Indicators: Crisis triggers: Tactics:	Indicators: Triggers: Tactics:
Communications and community infrastructure	Indicators: Triggers: Tactics:	Indicators: Crisis triggers: Tactics:	Indicators: Triggers: Tactics:
Staff	Indicators: Triggers: Tactics:	Indicators: Crisis triggers: Tactics:	Indicators: Triggers: Tactics:
Space/infrastructure	Indicators: Triggers: Tactics:	Indicators: Crisis triggers: Tactics:	Indicators: Triggers: Tactics:
Supplies	Indicators: Triggers: Tactics:	Indicators: Crisis triggers: Tactics:	Indicators: Triggers: Tactics:
Other categories	Indicators: Triggers: Tactics:	Indicators: Crisis triggers: Tactics:	Indicators: Triggers: Tactics:

REFERENCE

IOM (Institute of Medicine). 2012. *Crisis standards of care: A systems framework for catastrophic disaster response.* Washington, DC: The National Academies Press. http://www.nap.edu/openbook.php?record_id=13351 (accessed April 3, 2013).

6: Toolkit Part 2: Behavioral Health

INTRODUCTION

This chapter presents a discussion and decision-support tool to facilitate the development of indicators and triggers that help guide decision making about behavioral health during a disaster. Because integrated planning across the emergency response system is critical for a coordinated response, it is important to first read the introduction to the toolkit and materials relevant to the entire emergency response system in Chapter 3. Reviewing the toolkit chapters focused on other stakeholders would also be helpful.

Behavioral health is a term encompassing many topics. While there is growing use of and consensus on the term's application and meaning, there is also some inconsistency in its use and meaning. For the purposes of this document, behavioral health is intended to include factors related to overall psychological, psychiatric, and psychosocial healthiness and well-being. It also refers to specific psychiatric and substance abuse disorders.

Behavioral health is a pervasive factor affecting the response capabilities of decision makers and response personnel. It also affects the survival capabilities of the general public and those persons who require either acute or longer-term behavioral health treatment. Each of these groups faces common challenges in extreme events as well as unique stressors and intervention needs and opportunities.

It is important to highlight the centrality of understanding and attending to the sometimes unique needs of those whose roles include administration of, and response to, an extreme event. If the health of those involved (including behavioral health) is impacted in ways that adversely impact role function, the entire response can become compromised and, in extreme cases, fail. Preparedness activities must include detailed and strategic planning, which anticipates and addresses behavioral health consequences for both decision makers and responders. Preparedness activities should address issues such as strategies for identification, monitoring, and interventions geared toward stress reduction and management, as well as post-recovery resilience promotion and mitigation of posttraumatic stress disorder.

During an emergency, communities are confronted with a surge in demand and need for behavioral health intervention in health care facilities, in sheltering sites, at numerous public and private outpatient care venues, and through risk and crisis messaging and communications. When local health care capacity is being stretched beyond conventional care standards, the need for behavioral health alternative care strategies becomes essential either as an adjunct to general health care treatment or as a primary intervention for major behavioral health conditions (including substance abuse and addictive disorders).

Nobody who experiences a crisis (e.g., one described by scenarios provided) is unaffected by its psychosocial impact. The individual and collective impact will introduce considerable variability in people's ability to function. Behavioral health sequelae will impact the function of leaders, providers, and victims on both individual and collective levels. Understanding, anticipating, and specifically planning for these impacts is central to protection and promotion of the public's health and successful event and recovery management.

Discussions within local communities that include the widest array of stakeholders with the goal of planning alternatives to conventional care and preparing for the eventuality of providing only crisis care can mitigate the premature and/or inappropriate movement to this level of care through a proactive planning and resource allocation process. The recognition and inclusion of behavioral health stakeholders and factors in these complex decisions is an essential component of sound preparedness, response, and recovery.

Roles and Responsibilities

In the broadest sense, nearly every organization and system and every governmental level has a stake in ensuring efficacious response to behavioral health factors in large-scale emergencies and disasters. Addressing adverse impacts of stress, suggesting actions, and implementing strategies that promote resilience, and ensuring efforts that provide appropriate care of those with behavioral health disorders, is in everybody's best interest. Additional discussion about behavioral health in planning for and implementing crisis standards of care (CSC) is available in the Institute of Medicine's (IOM's) 2012 report *Crisis Standards of Care: A Systems Framework for Catastrophic Disaster Response.*

Special Circumstances

All extreme events require understanding of, and adaptation to, new and complex challenges. All of these challenges have behavioral health (as defined earlier in this chapter) elements. While all extreme events are stressful and demanding, some are especially difficult and complex. In these types of events, it is especially important that planners and incident leaders/managers understand the special psychosocial sequelae involved and ensure that behavioral health content experts are fully integrated into both decision making and response implementation. These include

- *Situations where a transition must be made in the fair and just allocation of resources and care when circumstances will not allow for the optimal level of care for all:* These are among the most difficult challenges that health care professionals can face. These are extraordinarily complex and difficult decisions that not only involve ethical and legal factors but also have major psychological impact on those involved in these actions and choices. Planners are strongly encouraged to involve behavioral health professionals in preparing for and implementing these difficult transitions. Integrating behavioral health consultation and services into this process will enhance the probability that adverse psychological consequences for those involved can be reduced.

- *Situations resulting in large-scale incapacitation or death of health care workers:* These situations not only degrade the capacity and capability of the health care system, they often bring grief and bereavement to remaining colleagues and coworkers. The result may increase the need for support services (including behavioral health) and result in performance problems in workers.
- *Events producing extremely large numbers of fatalities:* These events (especially with special circumstances; e.g., contaminated, partial, unidentifiable, or difficult-to-retrieve remains) create special challenges. Although these regrettable circumstances may actually result in low use of prehospital and hospital care, they frequently result in a significant expansion of behavioral health issues and needs.
- *Events resulting in potential long-term or unknown health consequences:* Events resulting in these types of health consequences can have a long-term impact on not only the medical status but also the psychosocial well-being of both workers and the general population.
- *Death or incapacity of key leaders and/or decision makers:* Sound disaster and emergency preparedness and response rely heavily on capable and trusted leadership. In the event these leaders are unable to play their important roles, the entire response will likely be compromised. In preparing for these events it is critical that strategies be developed and implemented that anticipate absent and/or impaired (including psychological) leadership.
- *Events evoking extreme emotions:* While all disasters provoke significant emotional responses in many, if not most, of those who experience them, some events evoke extreme emotions in large numbers of people. These reactions can have a significant impact on the health system (including behavioral health). As an example, some types of events can produce widespread rage. These events may include terrorism, violence disproportionately impacting the most vulnerable (e.g., children), and perceived social injustice. Planners should include these types of events and their impact on the public's health in their preparedness activities.

Because panic is so widely misunderstood, a brief discussion about it may be helpful. Panic is defined as behavior in which individuals and groups engage in actions that are motivated exclusively by self-preservation, even at the expense of the health, safety, and lives of others. Issues about panic in extreme events are often not well understood. Inaccurate assumptions sometimes lead to compromised preparedness and response efforts. While panic does occur, it is extremely rare. Several conditions are typically present in those rare instances where panic does appear. These include imminent threat to life, novelty of the situation, absence of leadership and/or authority, and extremely limited or nonexistent behavioral options. Planners should challenge assumptions that panic is a common, widespread, and easily triggered phenomenon. Planning should include strategies to address conditions where panic may occur, but recognize that it is far less common than is often assumed.

DISCUSSION AND DECISION-SUPPORT TOOL

Building on the scenarios and overarching key questions presented in Chapter 3, this tool contains additional questions to help participants drill down on the key issues and details for behavioral health. It also contains a chart that provides example behavioral health indicators, triggers, and tactics, and a blank chart for participants to complete. The scenarios, questions, and example chart are intended to provoke discussion that will help participants fill in the blank chart for their own situation.[1] Participants may choose to complete a single, general blank chart, or one each for various scenarios from their Hazard Vulnerability Analysis.

Discussion Participants and Key Stakeholders

Suggested participants and key stakeholders for a discussion focused on behavioral health are listed below.

- State and local public health agencies;
- State disaster medical advisory committee;
- State and local emergency medical services agencies;
- State and local emergency management agencies;
- Health care coalitions (HCCs), and where appropriate, U.S. Department of Veterans Affairs Medical Centers (VAMCs) and military treatment facilities (MTFs) that are part of those HCCs;
- State associations, including hospital, long-term care, home health, palliative care/hospice, and those that would reach private practitioners and other community-based providers;
- State and local law enforcement agencies;
- State and local elected officials;
- Representatives of key systems and stakeholders where changes in medical and public health (including behavioral health) status might present (e.g., large employers, primary and secondary schools, colleges and universities), law enforcement;
- Senior agency representatives for at-risk and vulnerable populations, such as persons with developmental disabilities, elder affairs, children and families, persons with acute and chronic behavioral health disorders, and developmental disabilities;
- Behavioral health practitioner associations and related licensing and regulatory boards;
- Members of the faith-based sheltering network and representatives of the behavioral health advocacy community, including, for example, Mental Health America and National Alliance on Mental Health, child/family advocacy groups, and the addiction recovery community;
- Behavioral health crisis response agencies tasked with operating various aspects of the community crisis response operations: (1) crisis lines, (2) mobile crisis teams that conduct face-to-face assessments, and (3) non-hospital-based crisis stabilization programs; and
- Additional nongovernmental agencies that could include chemical dependency recovery programs, methadone clinics, domestic abuse/sheltering agencies, and certified psychological first aid provider agencies.

---

[1] The blank table for participants to complete can be downloaded from the project's website: www.iom.edu/crisisstandards.

Key Questions: Slow-Onset Scenario

The questions below focus on the slow-onset influenza pandemic scenario presented in Chapter 3.[2]

Assumptions for Responding to a Slow-Onset Event

The gradual-onset pandemic scenario presents a complex set of behavioral health issues. The pre-event readiness planning process activated preparedness structures addressing ethical, legal, public health emergency management, and public stakeholder/advocacy concerns and responsibilities. The medical advisory committee (critical care, emergency department physicians, infectious disease and pediatric specialists) established guidelines (indicators and triggers) necessary to ethically and legally move from conventional standards of care to contingency and ultimately to CSC. Each developing phase of the pandemic, starting with pre-event planning, the onset of the event, the initiation of emergency operations, monitoring of the event features, and ongoing situational awareness, is accompanied by a corresponding degree of behavioral health assessment and intervention. The emerging discrepancy between behavioral health response capabilities and increasing demand from providers, patients/families, and the general public correspond directly with the intensity and complexity of the disaster event. The behavioral health discussion will need to address the crosscutting issues and population needs before, during, and after the event. The five key elements of ethical grounding, community and provider involvement, legal authority, clearly specified indicators, triggers and lines of responsibility, and the provision of evidence-based interventions are applicable to the development of CSC for behavioral health.

Key Questions[3]

1. Has the specificity of the Concept of behavioral health Operations integrated into command and response structures been tested?
2. What are the specific capabilities and capacities required for patients and families?
3. What are the specific capabilities and capacities required for providers?
4. What are the specific capabilities and capacities required for the general public?
5. What is necessary for rapid triage assessment and self-assessment behavioral health triage?
6. What is the continuum of acute behavioral health interventions needed?
7. What is the continuum of acute behavioral health interventions available?
8. What is the behavioral health risk/crisis communications strategic plan for each phase of the event?
9. What is the plan for postevent gap analysis to determine short-term strategies to meet additional behavioral health demand for services?
10. What is the strategy for building and sustaining health care provider resilience for all phases of the event?
11. What epidemiological surveillance capabilities and indicators require monitoring of behavioral health factors?

---

[2] These questions are provided to help start discussion; additional important questions may arise during the course of discussion. The questions are aimed at raising issues related to indicators and triggers, and are not comprehensive of all important questions related to disaster preparedness and response.

[3] Some of these questions are derived from Box 4-4 of IOM (2012, p. 1-90).

Key Questions: No-Notice Scenario

The questions below focus on the no-notice earthquake scenario presented in Chapter 3.

Assumptions for Responding to a Rapid-Onset Event

A rapid-onset event assumes immediate and massive destruction of the physical infrastructure and significant injury and loss of life to the general population within the incident area. The behavioral health impact is immediate and pervasive throughout the general population and the immediate responder community (also part of the general population). No-notice catastrophic events require strategies for addressing immediate loss of pre-event treatment capacity and accommodating mass fatalities and injury throughout the general population. Postincident trauma involves acute traumatic stress reactions throughout the responder and general population affecting all response capacity in the community. Activation and reassignment of behavioral health staff from non-impacted areas should be an integral feature of any initial (72-hour) response plan.

Key Questions

1. What behavioral health response strategy/resources can be deployed immediately and in 24-hour increments for the initial 72-hour postincident response period?
2. What specific actions should a hospital take to manage a surge involving both injured and uninjured (seeking information/bereaved) citizens?
3. Is/how is assessment of first responder capacity and fitness for duty (both physical and behavioral health) occurring?
4. Are triage strategies for the general population and delivery of low-level calming interventions in place?
5. What are the strategies for inpatient and residential behavioral health population evacuation? Are these strategies integrated with strategies of other required systems? What considerations have been made for the evacuation of the behavioral health population that receives care from community providers?
6. How is the first responder stress management cadre staffed and deployed?
7. How is surveillance of alternate care and sheltering sites for surge in demand for behavioral health intervention accomplished?
8. What are the strategies for treating widespread addiction/withdrawal?
9. What is the continuum of acute behavioral health interventions needed?
10. Is a behavioral health risk/crisis communications strategic plan in place for each phase of the event? Is there a strategy to have behavioral health input into risk/crisis communications of other stakeholders (e.g., public health, political leadership)?
11. What is the plan for postevent gap analysis to determine short-term strategies to meet additional behavioral health demand for services?
12. What is the strategy for building and sustaining health care provider resilience for all phases of the event?
13. What epidemiological surveillance capabilities and indicators require monitoring?
14. Has a disaster crisis line been activated and contact information published through traditional and other social media outlets?

Decision-Support Tool: Example Table

The indicators, triggers, and tactics shown in Table 6-1 are examples to help promote discussion and provide a sense of the level of detail and concreteness that is needed to develop useful indicators and triggers for a specific organization/agency/jurisdiction; they are not intended to be exhaustive or universally applicable. Prompted by discussion of the key questions above, discussion participants should fill out a blank table, focusing on key system indicators and triggers that will drive actions in their own organizations, agencies, and jurisdictions. As a reminder, *indicators* are measures or predictors of changes in demand and/or resource availability; *triggers* are decision points (refer back to the toolkit introduction [Chapter 3] for key definitions and concepts).

The example triggers shown in the table mainly are ones in which a "bright line" distinguishes functionally different levels of care (conventional, contingency, crisis). Because of the nature of this type of trigger, they can be described more concretely and can be included in a bulleted list. It is important to recognize, however, that expert analysis of one or more indicators may also trigger implementation of key response plans, actions, and tactics. This may be particularly true in a slow-onset scenario. In all cases, but particularly in the absence of bright lines, decisions may need to be made to *anticipate* upcoming problems and the implementation of tactics and to *lean forward* by implementing certain tactics before reaching the bright line or when no such line exists. These decision points vary according to the situation and are based on analysis, multiple inputs, recommendations, and, in certain circumstances, previous experience. Discussions about these tables should cover *how* such decisions would be made, even if the specifics cannot be included in a bulleted list in advance.

Note: (SO) designates indicators, triggers, and tactics that are most relevant to slow-onset scenarios, and (NN) designates indicators, triggers, and tactics that are most relevant to no-notice scenarios. Indicators, triggers, and tactics without such a marking are relevant to both no-notice and slow-onset scenarios.

TABLE 6-1
Example Behavioral Health (BH) Indicators, Triggers, and Tactics for Transitions Along the Continuum of Care

Indicator Category	Contingency	Crisis	Return Toward Conventional
Surveillance data: Community indicators	**Indicators** • Widespread acute anxiety and agitation increases presentations for treatment to and beyond normal limits • Hospitals experience a surge of not only medical patients, but searching family members; increased calls to hospitals as more people search for missing family members (NN) • Police, social services, schools, and others report increasing incidents of disruptive/ anxiety-driven behaviors (e.g., civil unrest and domestic violence, driving under the influence, etc.) • Increased psychiatric presentations in emergency department (ED) • Increased calls to BH-related crisis lines (e.g., suicide, domestic abuse, etc.) • Increased waiting list for appointments in BH providers • Hospitals begin to prematurely discharge BH patients (e.g., psychiatric, detox) **Triggers:** • X% increase in law enforcement/social services reports • Jail and alternative diversion programs are at capacity • X% increased psychiatric presentations in ED • X% increased calls to BH crisis lines • X% increased waiting list for appointments in BH providers • X% of BH providers report seeing only emergency cases **Tactics:** • Implement and expand early BH intervention strategies (e.g., psychological first aid, or PFA) • Implement/expand strategies to enhance crisis leadership • Increase overtime shifts for existing staff • Appropriately adjust and implement comprehensive risk/crisis communication strategies	**Indicators** • All data indicate continuing and increasing demand for BH-related services • Hospital services become increasingly compromised as a result of demands of searching family members (NN) • BH service providers are at capacity and refuse to take on new cases • Increased public presentation of BH casualties (e.g., overtly psychotic citizens, people ill from detox, increased drug-related crimes, etc.) • Widespread acute anxiety, agitation, and demand for care threaten integrity of treatment systems/sites • Alternative care/diversion programs (e.g., domestic violence shelters) are at capacity and cannot admit more • Jails are at capacity **Crisis Triggers:** • HCOs report that they can no longer admit patients exhibiting acute anxiety and agitation • Roads become impassable as a result of citizens evacuating and searching for members (NN) • EDs threaten closure because of inability to manage BH-related cases (e.g., no beds, no referral options) **Tactics:** • Implement a variety of local mutual aid agreements and federal disaster medical assistance teams and National Disaster Medical System resources (NN) • Diversion of psychiatric patients • Seek funding and other resources including government and refer to Disaster Medical Response Units (DMRUs) and medical special needs shelters • Route calls searching for missing family members to disaster hotline	**Indicators** • Decline in demands for services • Reduction of waiting lists to preevent levels • Number and severity of "new" cases declines • Reduced reports from police, social services, schools, and others regarding BH issues **Triggers:** • X% decline in demands for services • Reduction of waiting lists to pre-event levels • X% decline in number and severity of "new" cases • X% reduction in reports from law enforcement, social services, schools, and others regarding BH issues • Pre-event BH service capacity reestablished **Tactics:** • Continue and enhance monitoring of BH issues and service needs • Identify areas and/or populations with different patterns of recovery

- Seek and expand temporary employment of workers (including retirees, former employees, etc.)
- Implement health care organization (HCO) plan to cope with surge, sort BH and other health issues, and support staff and searching family members (NN)
- Route calls searching for missing family members to disaster hotline
- Transfer patients to alternative psychiatric and correctional sites designated for disaster response (SO)
- Expand sheltering and treatment capacity of state hospitals for civil and forensic patients (SO)

Community and communications infrastructure

Indicators:
- Families cannot find their loved ones (NN)
- Family members are separated (e.g., in different locations at time of earthquake or transported to different treatment sites) (NN)
- As a result of building damage, transportation system degradation, and communications systems failure, the population is unable to gather for support and ceremonies (NN)
- Communication mechanisms are degraded or nonexistent (NN)
- Other utilities (e.g., water, electricity) are degraded or nonexistent (NN)
- Roads and systems are becoming overloaded as a result of families trying to find their members (NN)
- Road congestion is complicated by arriving emergency vehicles from other jurisdictions (NN)
- General services are compromised and goods are in short supply, causing increased anxiety and agitation
- BH providers report delays and short supplies of prescription medication (e.g., antipsychotic, methadone, antidepression) because of supply line disruption
- Agitation increases as many/most basic community services are compromised
- Workplaces and schools close; status of persons in those structures unknown (NN)
- Work and school logistics become increasingly complex as schedules adapt to impact of event (causing increased fatigue and agitation) (SO)

Indicators:
- Road congestion becomes increasingly acute (NN)
- All data indicate continuing and increasing demand for BH-related services
- BH service providers are at capacity or have compromised facilities and refuse to take on new cases
- Increased public presentation of BH casualties (e.g., overtly psychotic citizens, people ill from detox, increased drug-related crimes, etc.)
- X% of workplaces and schools are closed (NN)
- Workplaces and schools report X% increases in lateness/absenteeism and decreases in productivity resulting from infrastructure degradation (SO)

Crisis triggers:
- HCOs report that they can no longer admit patients exhibiting acute anxiety and agitation
- Alternative care/diversion programs (e.g., domestic violence shelters) are at capacity and cannot admit more
- BH providers report they can no longer provide prescription medication (e.g., antipsychotic, methadone, antidepression) because of supply line disruption
- Widespread acute anxiety, agitation, and demand for care threaten integrity of treatment systems/sites

Indicators:
- Restoration of public services

Triggers:
- Acute anxiety, agitation, and demand for care no longer threaten integrity of treatment systems/sites

Tactics:
- Continue and enhance monitoring of BH issues and service needs
- Identify areas of infrastructure improvement and degradation
- Identify populations with different patterns of recovery and different infrastructure challenges

continued

TABLE 6-1
Continued

Indicator Category	Contingency	Crisis	Return Toward Conventional
Community and communications infrastructure (continued)	• Agitation increases as mail is delayed, automated teller machines are not replenished, etc. **Triggers:** • HCOs report that they can no longer admit patients exhibiting acute anxiety and agitation • Alternative care resources and diversion-receiving facilities are at capacity and cannot admit more • EDs threaten closure because of inability to manage BH-related cases (e.g., no beds, not referral options) • Jails are damaged and/or at capacity • Crisis phone lines and hotlines are disrupted • Forensic psychiatric unit is severely damaged; there is an immediate need to treat injured patients and evacuate others (NN) • Treatment facilities are damaged; extent of damage and continued use is unclear (NN) **Tactics:** • Implement risk/crisis communications strategies to inform, comfort, and reassure the public • Implement strategies for alternative sources for, and reallocation of, prescription medications • Monitor and prioritize infrastructure and supply degradation for early identification and anticipatory response • Identify regional facilities or temporary facilities that can provide capacity	**Tactics:** • Expand mutual aid arrangements for BH medications and staff • Expand work-from-home programs (SO) • Seek funding and other resources, including government • Implement alternative internal and response-related communication protocols (NN)	
Staff *[Refer also to the worker functional capacity table in Toolkit Part 1 (Table 3-1)]*	**Indicators:** • Staff are also earthquake victims; their ability to report to work is unclear (NN) • Requests for evaluations and services from BH staff increase • Requests from ED for BH specialty care (e.g., children, etc.) begin to increase • Increased frequency of psychological stress responses among health workforce (e.g., distractibility, hostility, hypervigilance, emotional extremes, interpersonal conflicts, etc.) • Increased absenteeism/presenteeism of critical staff persons	**Indicators:** • Requests to BH staff for patient evaluations and services approach capacity • Requests for BH specialty care (e.g., children, etc.) approach capacity • Frequency and severity of psychological stress responses among health workforce (e.g., distractibility, hostility, hypervigilance, emotional extremes, interpersonal conflicts, etc.) compromise patient care • Frequency and severity of psychological stress responses among health workforce compromise relationships among staff at any or all levels within the organization	**Indicators:** • BH staff become more able to provide patient evaluations and services • Availability of BH specialty care (e.g., children, etc.) begins to return toward baseline • Staff resources increase and exhausted staff are able to rotate out of deployment

- Increased demands on employee assistance programs (EAPs); private BH practitioners are not readily available (SO)
- Increases in requests for psychological fitness for duty assessments of staff
- Increased reports of stress-related sequelae in other systems (e.g., law enforcement, social services, faith organizations, etc.)

Triggers:
- Requests to BH staff for patient evaluations and services increase by X%
- Requests for BH specialty care (e.g., children, etc.) increase by X%
- X% increase in staff absenteeism (NN)/presenteeism (SO)
- X% increases in frequency of psychological stress responses among health workforce (e.g., distractibility, hostility, hypervigilance, emotional extremes, interpersonal conflicts, unscheduled time away from duty station, increased demand for stress management support, etc.)
- X% increase in demands on EAPs
- X% increases in requests for psychological fitness for duty assessments of staff
- X% increase in informal personnel complaints

Tactics:
- Implement and expand early BH intervention strategies (e.g., PFA)
- Implement/expand strategies to enhance crisis leadership
- Implement expanded and alternative ways to establish and maintain contact with staff (NN)
- If possible explore and establish a means for staff families to be housed and supported at HCO (NN)
- Appropriately adjust and implement comprehensive risk/crisis communication strategies
- Expand temporary employment of workers (including retired, former employees, etc.)
- Review and appropriately modify personnel policies and practices where possible
- Assess the potential to obtain or enhance specialized consultation in areas of workplace stress and disaster BH
- Mobilize stress management team for responders and staff

- Absenteeism/presenteeism compromises patient care and/or organizational function
- EAP resources approach capacity
- Requests for psychological fitness for duty assessments of staff approach capacity to process
- Increasing reports of stress-related sequelae in other systems (e.g., law enforcement, social services, faith organizations, etc.), school, employers (SO)

Crisis triggers:
- Requests to BH staff for patient evaluations and services reach capacity and no additional service can be provided
- Existing services cannot be maintained
- Requests for BH specialty care (e.g., children, etc.) can no longer be fulfilled
- Absenteeism/presenteeism causes shutdown of services
- EAPs can no longer accept new referrals and/or manage existing caseloads
- Requests for psychological fitness for duty assessments of staff increase to a level where they cannot be processed in a timely/quality manner
- Increase in formal personnel complaints cannot be processed in a timely/quality manner

Tactics:
- Implement and expand early BH intervention strategies (e.g., PFA)
- Implement or expand strategies to support leadership
- Appropriately adjust and implement comprehensive risk/crisis communication strategies
- Seek to expand temporary employment of workers (including retired, former employees, etc.)
- Review and appropriately modify personnel policies and practices where possible
- Assess the potential to obtain or enhance specialized consultation in areas of workplace stress and disaster BH
- Implement mutual aid and other resource enhancement strategies
- Mobilize stress management team for responders and staff (NN)

- Frequency and severity of psychological stress responses among health workforce allows for resumption of routine staffing ratios
- Absenteeism/presenteeism declines
- Requests for psychological fitness-for-duty assessments of staff decline
- Reports of stress-related sequelae in other systems (e.g., law enforcement, schools, employers, etc.) decline

Triggers:
- BH staff are able to meet needs for patient evaluations and services
- Reduction in absenteeism/presenteeism to level where services begin functioning
- EAPs begin to accept new referrals and/or can now manage existing caseloads
- Requests for psychological fitness for duty assessments of staff decrease to baseline and can be processed in a timely/quality manner
- Decrease in formal personnel complaints/litigation to baseline and can be processed in a timely/quality manner

continued

TABLE 6-1
Continued

Indicator Category	Contingency	Crisis	Return Toward Conventional
Space/infrastructure	**Indicators:** • Specialty psychiatric units experience increased use • Specialty psychiatric units experience damage and must treat injured and/or consider evacuation (NN) • Hospital triage results in BH (e.g., psychiatric, detox) patients being discharged before scheduled • Health care facilities initiate alternative space use plans to accommodate additional beds and space for families • Increases in service provision/consultation in ways other than face to face • Social distancing reduces support for patients, families, community (SO) **Triggers:** • Specialty psychiatric units exceed capacity • Hospital triage results in BH patients being discharged before scheduled **Tactics:** • Increase alternate care sites/services for BH patients • Increase surveillance of BH needs and resources across systems • Update mutual aid strategies/plans • Update plans and strategies for obtaining outside BH or other help • Refer to DMRUs and medical special needs shelters (NN)	**Indicators:** • Specialty psychiatric units exceed capacity • Specialty psychiatric units experience damage and must treat injured and/or the decision is made to evacuate (NN) • Hospital triage results in reduction of BH (e.g., psychiatric, detox) patients admitted (NN) • Increased numbers of BH patients being maintained in ED or general medical treatment areas • Very heavy use of service provision/consultation in ways other than face to face • BH problems increase in hospitals as patient families, searching family members, and bereaved family members share space and services (NN) • Increasing BH problems resulting from social distancing (e.g., depression, suicide, substance abuse, etc.) (SO) **Crisis triggers:** • Specialty psychiatric units not available and unable to safely board in ED or other locations • Alternative BH treatment sites/services are at capacity • BH patients can no longer be maintained in ED or general medical treatment areas • Most service provision/consultation occurs in ways other than face to face • BH problems compromise function/services in hospitals as patient families, searching family members, and bereaved family members share space and services; key hospital resources are redirected to manage the situation (NN) • Pervasive BH problems resulting from social distancing (e.g., depression, suicide, substance abuse, etc.) (SO) **Tactics:** • Increase surveillance of BH needs and resources across systems • Update mutual aid strategies/plans • Activate plans and strategies for obtaining outside BH or other help	**Indicators:** • Specialty psychiatric units are no longer at capacity • Admission of and services to BH (e.g., psychiatric, detox) patients admitted increases (NOTE: This marker of recovery involves increasing admits because it is *relative to the ability to admit* vs. prior lack of beds.) • Decreasing numbers of BH patients being maintained in ED or general medical treatment areas • Health care facilities require less alternative space usage, freeing up beds for BH patients • Care and consultation again begin to occur face to face • Decreasing BH problems resulting from social distancing (e.g., depression, suicide, substance abuse, etc.)/less social distancing **Triggers:** • Specialty psychiatric units admissions and census return to baseline • Admission of and services to BH (e.g., psychiatric, detox) patients returns to baseline • BH patients being maintained in ED or general medical treatment areas returns to baseline **Tactics:** • Maintain/increase surveillance of BH needs and resources across systems • Deactivate incident-specific hotlines and alternate care spaces • Activate plans and strategies for release or return of outside BH or other help

Indicators:

- Demand increases for psychiatric medications and medications used to treat substance abuse disorders
- Supply of psychiatric medications and medications used to treat substance abuse disorders decreases
- Patients have lost their prescriptions/medications in the earthquake or are unable to access them (NN)
- Remaining functioning pharmacies have limited computer capacity to confirm prescription status (NN)
- Reports of self-medication increase
- Increasing numbers of patients begin to experience/exhibit withdrawal symptoms

Triggers:

- Demand for psychiatric medications and medications used to treat substance abuse disorders increases by X%
- X% reduction in supply of psychiatric medications and medications used to treat substance abuse disorders
- X% increase in numbers of behaviorally agitated patient requests for detox services for withdrawal symptoms of any type (from a wide variety of licit and illicit drugs)

Tactics:

- Increase monitoring of supply and demand for BH-related medications
- Implement strategies to optimize efficiency of supply lines/processes
- Explore alternative supply lines and processes to ensure medication availability
- Circulate guidance on alternative medications, dangers of self-dosing, and resources for help/detox

Indicators:

- Demand or projected demand for psychiatric medications and medications used to treat substance abuse disorders exceeds supply
- Supply of psychiatric medications and medications used to treat substance abuse disorders decreases to the point of limited medication provision
- Self-medication becomes a significant factor in large numbers of law enforcement, emergency medical services (EMS), hospital encounters
- Health care organizations are referring increasing numbers of patients experiencing/exhibiting withdrawal symptoms

Crisis triggers:

- Key psychiatric and substance abuse treatment medications are no longer available
- Self-medication becomes a significant factor in large numbers of law enforcement and health care organization encounters and compromises systems function (e.g., adverse impact on worker productivity, high demand for medical intervention, increased costs, etc.)

Tactics:

- Increase monitoring of supply and demand for BH-related medications
- Implement strategies to optimize efficiency of supply lines/processes
- Implement alternative supply lines processes to ensure medication availability
- Implement BH patient evacuation to out-of-state hospitals (SO)
- Recommend triage strategies and dosing strategies to address critical shortages

Indicators:

- Demand for psychiatric medications and medications used to treat substance abuse disorders and is returning toward baseline
- Supply of psychiatric medications and medications used to treat substance abuse disorders increases
- Self-medication becomes a declining factor in law enforcement, HCO encounters
- HCOs see a declining number of patients experiencing/exhibiting withdrawal symptoms

Triggers:

- Demand for psychiatric medications and medications used to treat substance abuse disorders returns to baseline
- Supply of psychiatric medications and medications used to treat substance abuse disorders adequate to meet community needs
- HCOs see a return to baseline in the number of patients experiencing/exhibiting withdrawal symptoms

Tactics:

- Continue/improve monitoring of supply and demand for BH-related medications
- Evaluate efficacy of strategies to optimize efficiency of supply lines/processes
- Review and revise recommendations for medication use/triage

continued

TABLE 6-1
Continued

Indicator Category	Contingency	Crisis	Return Toward Conventional
Other categories: **Fatality management**	**Indicators:** • Hospital and civic morgues approach capacity • Community distress over visible disinterment in local cemeteries (NN) • Death becomes an increasing topic in conversation, media, and public meetings • Recovered remains are partial, creating increased stress on workers, families (NN) • It becomes increasingly clear that body recovery will be a protracted process, increasing stress on workers and families (NN) • Citizens are increasingly agitated because of delays in issuance of death certificates and resulting inability to obtain survivor benefits and services **Triggers:** • Community experiences mass fatalities in a very short period of time • Death-related supplies are increasingly difficult to obtain (e.g., body bags, caskets, etc.) • Burials are delayed **Tactics:** • Review mass fatality plans • Seek advice from BH bereavement specialists, disaster mortuary operational response teams (DMORTs), faith community, other experienced sources • Review and provide risk/crisis communication training • Convene stakeholders on a regular basis to monitor and assess trends/issues	**Indicators:** • Death rate continues unabated or increases • The population is unable to gather for support and ceremonies because of contagion • Hospital and civic morgues are at or over capacity • Death dominates conversation, media, and public meetings • Delayed recovery, including decomposition of remains, increases stress for workers and families (NN) **Crisis triggers:** • Temporary interment and "unofficial" burials occurring or considered • Death-related supplies cannot be obtained (e.g., body bags, caskets, etc.) • Storage of remains becomes a problem and temporary solutions are employed **Tactics:** • Implement and adapt mass fatality plans • Open family assistance center (NN) • Seek advice from BH bereavement specialists, DMORTs, faith community, other experienced sources • Expand risk/crisis communication training • Continue to convene stakeholders on a regular basis to monitor and assess trends/issues • Implement mutual aid (including temporary morgues) • Coordinate with faith-based and cultural advocacy groups to address concerns and manage expectations about burial options, processes, risks	**Indicators:** • Death rate declines • The population is increasingly able to gather for support and ceremonies • Death becomes less dominant in conversation, media, and public meeting • Burials are resuming; issues of storage of remains become less acute • Death certificate processing times are becoming shorter • Media sensational and provocative stories about bodies decline and are replaced with stories of survival, resilience, and moving forward **Triggers:** • Hospital and civic morgues can accommodate demand • Death-related supplies are more available (e.g., body bags, caskets, etc.) **Tactics:** • Evaluate and modify mass fatality plans • Update roster of BH bereavement specialists, DMORTS, faith community, other experienced sources • Enlist those who can help the community memorialize the event and its aftermath as a way of individual and collective healing • Expand and institutionalize risk/crisis communication training • Continue to convene stakeholders on a regular basis to monitor and assess trends/issues • Demobilize family assistance centers and other resources as appropriate

Other categories: Risk/crisis communications

Indicators:

- Key government officials refuse to make public statements
- "Experts" in media are increasing community fear/confusion/anger
- Racial and ethnic groups in the community are differentially affected or obtaining and understanding different information
- Rumors are growing
- There is inconsistency in health messages from various official sources
- Messaging is increasingly inconsistent with current standards of care and status of health system elements
- Issues of social justice, historical animosities, incapable leadership, etc., begin to increase in the media and at public events

Triggers:

- Event involves high degree of risk or concern (contagion, contamination, delayed effects)
- Public is demanding answers/reassurance/direction
- Media are providing inconsistent messaging

Tactics:

- Community leaders promoted as credible sources of information
- Review, update, and implement crisis communication plans
- Implement Joint Information System—develop, vet, and circulate press and information releases
- Proactively schedule briefings and make credible experts available
- Provide just-in-time crisis communication training for formal and informal leaders
- Seek specialized consultation and advice regarding risk/crisis communication
- Increase content monitoring and analysis of media (including social media) for tone, accuracy, usability, consistency
- Obtain information from nontraditional sources to determine how information is being provided/interpreted in vulnerable or specific cultural groups

Indicators:

- Public is increasingly insistent and angry at lack of direction and answers
- Media continue to provide inconsistent messaging even when provided with credible information
- Some community leaders are discredited as sources of information; they are marginalized and/or removed
- Key government officials continue to refuse to make public statements
- "Experts" in media are increasing community fear/confusion/anger; some come to the community and create increased disruption
- Racial and ethnic groups in the community are differentially affected or obtaining and understanding different information; talk of demonstrations and civil protest increases
- Rumors are growing
- There continues to be inconsistency in health messages from various official sources
- Messaging is increasingly inconsistent with current standards of care and status of health system elements
- Information is inaccurate and changing about locations for vaccinations, causing anger among the general population

Crisis triggers:

- Issues of social justice, historical animosities, incapable leadership, etc., dominate the media and public events
- Civil unrest occurs

Tactics:

- Aggressive implementation of crisis communication plans—additional resources for rumor control, specific population targeted messages, social media responses
- Provide just-in-time crisis communication training for formal and informal leaders
- Seek specialized consultation and advice regarding risk/crisis communication
- Increase content monitoring and analysis of media for tone, accuracy, usability, consistency

Indicators:

- Public is increasingly satisfied with information they are receiving; less public anger and frustration
- Emerging community leaders are solidified in their roles as credible sources of information
- Discredited leaders are seen and heard from less
- Key government officials increase public visibility and apply risk/communications training in their public statements
- The media are moving on to other stories and outside "experts" are seen less frequently; the community is increasingly perceived as able to handle challenges
- Different racial and ethnic groups in the community are increasingly getting the same credible information; talk of demonstrations and civil protest decreases
- Rumors are identified early and accurate information is effectively communicated

Triggers:

- Media are providing more consistent messaging and increasingly use credible information
- Consistency in health messages from various official sources increases
- Messaging more accurately reflects current standards of care and status of health system

Tactics:

- Evaluate and revise crisis communication plans
- Institutionalize crisis communication training for formal and informal leaders
- Update roster of specialized consultants/advisers in risk/crisis communication

continued

TABLE 6-1
Continued

Indicator Category	Contingency	Crisis	Return Toward Conventional
Other categories: Risk/crisis communications (continued)		• Deploy crisis counseling teams to health resource lines to address social unrest • Convene stakeholders regarding issues of, and strategies for, crisis communication • Focus on positive accomplishment or developments in communications • Meet with major media to emphasize gravity of situation and attempt to address conflicts in messaging	• Continue and enhance content monitoring and analysis of media for tone, accuracy, usability, consistency • Continue to convene stakeholders regarding issues of, and strategies for, crisis communication • Focus on positive accomplishments/developments • Continue to aggressively address rumors and monitor new developments

Decision-Support Tool: Blank Table to Be Completed

Prompted by discussion of the key questions above, participants should fill out this blank table (or multiple tables for different scenarios) with key system indicators and triggers that will drive actions in their own organizations, agencies, and jurisdictions.[4]

Reminders:

- *Indicators* are measures or predictors of changes in demand and/or resource availability; *triggers* are decision points.
- The key questions were designed to facilitate discussion—customized for behavioral health—about the following four steps to consider when developing indicators and triggers for a specific organization/agency/jurisdiction: (1) identify key response strategies and actions, (2) identify and examine potential indicators, (3) determine trigger points, and (4) determine tactics.
- Discussions about triggers should include (a) triggers for which a "bright line" can be described, and (b) *how* expert decisions to implement tactics would be made using one or more indicators for which no bright line exists. Discussions should consider the benefits of *anticipating* the implementation of tactics, and of *leaning forward* to implement certain tactics in advance of a bright line or when no such line exists.
- The example table may be consulted to promote discussion and to provide a sense of the level of detail and concreteness that is needed to develop useful indicators and triggers for a specific organization/agency/jurisdiction.
- This table is intended to frame discussions and create awareness of information, policy sources, and issues at the agency level to share with other stakeholders. Areas of uncertainty should be noted and clarified with partners.
- Refer back to the toolkit introduction (Chapter 3) for key definitions and concepts.

---

[4] The blank table for participants to complete can be downloaded from the project's website: www.iom.edu/crisisstandards.

Scope and Event Type: _____

Indicator Category	Contingency	Crisis	Return Toward Conventional
Surveillance data	Indicators: Triggers: Tactics:	Indicators: Crisis triggers: Tactics:	Indicators: Triggers: Tactics:
Communications and community infrastructure	Indicators: Triggers: Tactics:	Indicators: Crisis triggers: Tactics:	Indicators: Triggers: Tactics:
Staff	Indicators: Triggers: Tactics:	Indicators: Crisis triggers: Tactics:	Indicators: Triggers: Tactics:
Space/infrastructure	Indicators: Triggers: Tactics:	Indicators: Crisis triggers: Tactics:	Indicators: Triggers: Tactics:
Supplies	Indicators: Triggers: Tactics:	Indicators: Crisis triggers: Tactics:	Indicators: Triggers: Tactics:
Other categories	Indicators: Triggers: Tactics:	Indicators: Crisis triggers: Tactics:	Indicators: Triggers: Tactics:

REFERENCE

IOM (Institute of Medicine). 2012. *Crisis standards of care: A systems framework for catastrophic disaster response.* Washington, DC: The National Academies Press. http://www.nap.edu/openbook.php?record_id=13351 (accessed April 3, 2013).

7: Toolkit Part 2: Emergency Medical Services

INTRODUCTION

This chapter presents a discussion and decision-support tool to facilitate the development of indicators and triggers that help guide emergency medical services (EMS) decision making during a disaster. Because integrated planning across the emergency response system is critical for a coordinated response, it is important to first read the introduction to the toolkit and materials relevant to the entire emergency response system in Chapter 3. Reviewing the toolkit chapters focused on other stakeholders also would be helpful.

Roles and Responsibilities

The role and expanse of responsibilities of the EMS professional go far beyond prehospital patient care delivery and transport. Emergency medical dispatch (EMD) plays the critical role as the "gatekeeper" of the resources and assets that must be appropriately dispatched and distributed for a successful emergency response. Once on the scene, the EMS provider is the direct observant of the scene of the incident, if an accident, or of the patient's residence. It is often the EMS provider who notes that a patient may not have any or insufficient resources within his or her residence to maintain independence or personal safety. Therefore, an important message to include in any crisis planning is that all personnel, regardless of years of experience or expertise, should be (and feel) empowered to report any unusual events, observations on the scene, or surge in patient complaints or threats to an administrative avenue that is operational and responsive at all times.

The role of the EMS medical director is very important. This individual is a physician with a solid foundation of knowledge and expertise in emergency medical dispatch, EMS, emergency medicine, public health, triage, and appropriate allocation of resources who can serve in a leading role during an emergency or catastrophic incident. The continuous partnership of the EMS medical director with the EMS agency supervisor as a unified team during all aspects of the response cannot be understated.

Each state has the statutory authority and responsibility to regulate EMS within its borders. In addition, each state has the authority over the certification or licensure of their EMS providers, EMS scope of practice, and EMS provider titles. For the delivery of EMS services, some states have mandatory statewide protocols while others permit the use of variable regional or local protocols. During the creation of crisis standards of care (CSC) plans, the state EMS offices and the National Association of State EMS Officials

(NASEMSO), the lead national organization for state EMS offices, are invaluable assets. They are the best sources of EMS-specific information regarding individual state EMS system structure and state EMS administrative, legislative, and operational requirements and practices. During routine and evolving crises that will not require a federal response or gubernatorial declaration of emergency, the state EMS offices and NASEMSO are assets of knowledge and support. Special attention to neighboring state EMS systems must be consistently included at all levels of CSC because emergency dispatch and response, prehospital care delivery, and patient transport occur routinely across state lines on a daily basis during conventional levels of care in many jurisdictions.

Additional discussion about EMS roles and responsibilities in planning for and implementing CSC is available in the Institute of Medicine's (IOM's) 2012 report *Crisis Standards of Care: A Systems Framework for Catastrophic Disaster Response*. This report also includes planning and implementation templates that outline core functions and tasks.

Key Considerations for EMS

Disaster planning has been a core component for the EMS community for many years. As a result, EMS providers tend to have integrated adaptation skills in their routine practice. The concept of CSC, with the three stages of conventional, contingency, and crisis levels, is a relatively new concept for many in the health care community, including EMS providers. In the past, the focus has been on crisis planning rather than maximizing crucial tactics at the conventional and contingency phases to avoid entering a state of crisis.

This toolkit is designed to serve as a facilitator of creative, flexible, and expansive thought during the development of processes and protocols for the EMS disaster planning team. CSC require a shift from the former culture and mindset of disaster planning of a binary response (disaster or not) to a continuum of services that can be provided based on demand, with adaptations at each step to allow the system to bend, but not break. The EMS agency should craft its plan in a manner that best incorporates and coordinates the available local, regional, state, and federal resources into a framework that serves the jurisdiction. A disaster response team should have and be able to execute a plan to manage a response to victims without an adequate supply of medical resources. Such a team should have and be able to execute a plan to retain, secure, and maintain the EMS workforce instead of writing a plan where the primary focus is on managing a disaster without staffing.

Significant alterations in response procedures and allocation of resources may be required at the contingency level, with the primary goal of avoiding a transition into the crisis level. Important elements that must accompany these procedures include training and disaster exercises that actively include emergency medical dispatch, EMS, and EMS medical direction; community engagement and education; repeated and frequent dissemination of timely and accurate information to the community and the Joint Information Center; and appropriate regulatory relief and liability protection for the parameters included in both contingency and CSC. Ideally, these groups should be included in all disaster training exercises along with organizations in the private and public sectors and any out-of-state agencies that may be dispatched for mutual aid.

The true test of the fortitude of the EMD and EMS response system is to stress it beyond its capacity. The most valuable disaster exercises will tax this system beyond its limits and demonstrate how well the participants identify indicators, recognize critical triggers, and develop and implement adaptive and effective tactics. In the creation of disaster exercises as well as in conventional operations, it is beneficial for an EMS system to break down the barriers between public and private EMS agencies and cultivate symbiotic partnerships between these organizations. As a disaster transitions through the conventional, contingency, and crisis plans, there must also be triggers and indicators that signal the incident commander that the crisis is deescalating and potentially approaching resolution (though in long-term events, a return to conventional status may be only temporary). In partnership and close liaison with the emergency management system and other key emergency response system stakeholders, those with nimble minds who can create a path less trodden and use reduced resources effectively will be successful.

DISCUSSION AND DECISION-SUPPORT TOOL

Building on the scenarios and overarching key questions presented in Chapter 3, this tool contains additional questions to help participants drill down on the key issues and details for EMS. It also contains a chart that provides example EMS indicators, triggers, and tactics, and a blank chart for participants to complete. The scenarios, questions, and example chart are intended to provoke discussion that will help participants fill in the blank chart for their own agency.[1] Participants may choose to complete a single, general blank chart, or one each for various scenarios from their Hazard Vulnerability Analysis.

Discussion Participants

Suggested participants for a discussion focused on EMS are listed below.

- EMS agencies;
- EMS medical directors;
- Emergency medical dispatch centers;
- Call centers and medical resource control centers;
- Public and private prehospital transport agencies (including first response agencies);
- Local hospitals and long-term care facilities;
- Local public health agencies;[2]
- Local emergency management agencies;
- Mutual aid network participants;
- Local emergency planning committees;
- Public and private evacuation transportation partners;
- Local and regional medical supply agencies;
- Law enforcement agencies;
- Local or regional legal representative; and
- State EMS office liaison.

---

[1] The blank table for participants to complete can be downloaded from the project's website: www.iom.edu/crisisstandards.

[2] EMS frequently works with people with serious and persistent mental illness and substance abuse, even outside of disaster situations. Depending on local and state structures, behavioral health officials may be located in different agencies: for example, public health or health and human services. It will be important to engage them in the deliberative process, and to include consideration of behavioral health issues (see Chapter 6 for more details).

Key Emergency Response System Stakeholders

Suggested stakeholders for the EMS-focused discussion are listed below. These entities should be involved at some point in the deliberation process, although they may not participate in initial discussions because of the need to keep the group at a manageable size.

- State EMS offices;
- State emergency management agencies;
- State medical disaster committee;
- State EMS/trauma committees;
- State public health agencies;
- State hospital and long-term care associations;
- State trauma offices;
- State health and human services agencies;
- State law enforcement agencies;
- Regional and local EMS advisory councils;
- Regional and local health care coalitions;
- Regional and local trauma advisory councils;
- State and local disaster response network members; and
- Regional and local law enforcement agencies.

Key Questions: Slow-Onset Scenario

The questions below are focused on the slow-onset influenza pandemic scenario presented in Chapter 3:[3]

1. What information from dispatch centers would drive actions on this event? How is that information shared?
2. What information/trigger would alert EMS to take specific actions such as donning a higher level of personal protective equipment (PPE)?
3. What information from EMS agencies would be shared with local public health and when? How is that information conveyed?
4. What information from the hospitals or skilled nursing facilities regarding this type of event would determine the EMS system's actions? How is that information communicated to EMS?
5. What information is needed from public health regarding this type of event? How is that information obtained?
6. What guidelines and measures are in place to protect EMS personnel from becoming ill?
7. What actions can be taken if EMS agencies are unable to staff ambulances appropriately according to their usual model?

---

[3] These questions are provided to help start discussion; additional important questions may arise during the course of discussion. The questions are aimed at raising issues related to indicators and triggers, and are not comprehensive of all important questions related to disaster preparedness and response.

8. What precautions would be initiated to provide protection (physical [including PPE], mental, behavioral, etc.) to EMS personnel during this event?

9. What just-in-time training could be implemented when medications or equipment become scarce? How will these programs, along with the associated protocols, be disseminated and implemented?

10. What criteria would be used in the treatment of patients in this type of event?

11. What process should be implemented to change response and transport protocols within the organization and with state licensing agencies? What measures can be implemented if EMS agencies cannot transport patients to a health care organization?

12. How will EMS agencies respond to or triage calls if they have limited or no ambulances to transport patients?

13. What information needs to be known in order to return to contingency or conventional care?

14. What expanded role can EMS personnel provide in this type of event (EMS role at alternate care sites, vaccination sites, etc.)? Are protections in place for this expanded role? Are providers prepared to take on these responsibilities?

15. What should an EMS agency do if they have more patients to treat than they can manage?

16. At what point should an EMS agency go back to medical direction for additional medical oversight or changes to standard operating procedures (SOPs)? For example, at what point should ambulance staffing patterns be altered and normal scopes of practice expanded?

Key Questions: No-Notice Scenario

The questions below are focused on the no-notice earthquake scenario presented in Chapter 3:

1. What information does dispatch need to know to request mutual aid?

2. What information does EMS need to know from hospitals or other health care organizations? How will this information be communicated to EMS?

3. What information is needed from public health or emergency management that would drive actions on this event?

4. What information is needed to activate the EMS agency's mass casualty plan and request additional medical resources?

5. What information is needed and how does EMS incident command identify a potential need for a declaration of emergency for a mass casualty incident?

6. What should the EMS agency do if they have more patients than they can transport?

7. What should the EMS agency do if they have no more personnel to assist with triage and treatment?

8. When/how will existing trauma field triage criteria and associated destination protocols be modified or abandoned?

9. What just-in-time training could be implemented when medications or equipment become scarce? How will these programs, along with the associated protocols, be disseminated and implemented?

10. How will the EMS agency manage specialty care patients (e.g., burn, contaminated, pediatrics), particularly when usual referral centers are unavailable or unreachable?

11. What information (or permission) is needed to activate CSC plans?
12. How are incoming staff, equipment, and patient transport resources coordinated between jurisdictions?
13. What system status management information is available to determine indicators and triggers and how are they communicated to leadership and other emergency response systems organizations?
14. What triggers at the state level exist to provide regulatory and liability protection as well as additional resources? How does the EMS agency communicate needs and request these resources?

Decision-Support Tool: Example Table

The indicators, triggers, and tactics shown in Table 7-1 are examples to help promote discussion and provide a sense of the level of detail and concreteness that is needed to develop useful indicators and triggers for a specific organization/agency/jurisdiction; they are not intended to be exhaustive or universally applicable. Prompted by discussion of the key questions above, discussion participants should fill out a blank table, focusing on key system indicators and triggers that will drive actions in their own organizations, agencies, and jurisdictions. As a reminder: *indicators* are measures or predictors of changes in demand and/or resource availability; *triggers* are decision points (refer back to the toolkit introduction [Chapter 3] for key definitions and concepts).

The example triggers shown in Table 7-1 below mainly are ones in which a "bright line" distinguishes functionally different levels of care (conventional, contingency, crisis). Because of the nature of this type of trigger, they can be described more concretely and can be included in a bulleted list. It is important to recognize, however, that expert analysis of one or more indicators may also trigger implementation of key response plans, actions, and tactics. This may be particularly true in a slow-onset scenario. In all cases, but particularly in the absence of "bright lines," decisions may need to be made to *anticipate* upcoming problems and the implementation of tactics and to *lean forward* by implementing certain tactics before reaching the bright line or when no such line exists. These decision points vary according to the situation and are based on analysis of multiple inputs, recommendations, and, in certain circumstances, previous experience. Discussions about these tables should cover *how* such decisions would be made, even if the specifics cannot be included in a bulleted list in advance.

TABLE 7-1
Example Emergency Medical Services (EMS) Indicators, Triggers, and Tactics for Transitions Along the Continuum of Care

Indicator Category	Contingency	Crisis	Return Toward Conventional
Scope of the event	Minor or major disaster	Catastrophic	Approaching resolution
Surveillance data	**Indicators:** • Increased patient encounters by EMS • Increased emergency department and/or hospital census • Reports of increased cases of influenza • Reports of an earthquake with potential of additional aftershocks **Triggers:** • Significantly elevated number of dispatch requests • Significantly increased patient care encounters with similar signs and symptoms or high patient acuity • Significantly increased data registry entries from state or regional electronic prehospital patient care record systems **Tactics:** • Advise local health officials (or, as applicable, base station or online medical direction) of the observed increase in activity or increased incidence of patients with similar signs and symptoms • Establish incident command for EMS and advise the emergency care system stakeholders of this action command • Provide incident command with frequent reports and ongoing trends using surveillance data • Engage regional and state surveillance systems to follow trends and expanse of the mass casualty incident or pandemic • Engage mutual aid partners as required	**Indicators:** • Patient care demands exceed the available EMS resources, including mutual aid • Patient care demands exceed the available hospital resources • Confirmation of increased virulence of the strain of influenza • Surveillance data are impacted due to overwhelmed health care providers, public health, or collapse of data entry systems • The incidence of illness and injury continues to escalate despite mitigation measures **Crisis Triggers:** • Multiple hospitals closed to EMS • Mutual aid partners not able to answer calls involving potential life threats **Tactics:** • Maximize alternative avenues of data collection and submission (verbal, paper, or estimated reports) • Continue to advise local health officials (or, as applicable, base station or online medical direction) of the observed increase in activity or increased incidence of patients with similar signs and symptoms • Work with mutual aid agencies to revise and/or implement call triage	**Indicators:** • Stabilization or decrease in patient encounters by EMS • Stabilization or decrease in emergency department and/or hospital census • Stabilization or decrease in the reports of cases of influenza • Decreasing frequency of earthquake aftershocks **Triggers:** • Stabilization or decrease in the number of dispatch requests • Stabilization or decrease in calls with similar signs and symptoms or high patient acuity calls **Tactics:** • Monitor the surveillance data for resurgence or continued mitigation • Continue to advise local health officials (or, as applicable, base station or online medical direction) of the observed increase in activity or increased incidence of patients with similar signs and symptoms

continued

TABLE 7-1
Continued

Indicator Category	Contingency	Crisis	Return Toward Conventional
Community and communications infrastructure	**Indicators:** • Compromised communications (911, public safety) systems • Reports of widespread road or structural damage • Increased calls or ambulatory presentation of patients to EMS agencies seeking medical advice or treatment • Inaccurate information from unreliable sources circulating within the community **Triggers:** • >20% increase in emergency medical dispatch or medical advice hotlines • An increase in rumors and inaccurate information within the lay population, media, and social networking sites **Tactics:** • Initiate community education regarding selective emergency medical dispatch (EMD) and EMS triage and transport measures • Engage with media outlets to disseminate information on mitigation measures • Work with emergency management and crews in the field to obtain situational awareness regarding access and damage reports • Consider partnering to establish nurse call triage lines to mitigate requests for EMS transport	**Indicators:** • Emergency medical dispatch overwhelmed by call volumes and unable to answer all calls • 911 system compromised • Media reports that incite increased anxiety • Operational or structural collapse of the communication centers • Inaccurate information is in the forefront **Crisis Triggers:** • Inability of high-acuity patients to access the emergency response system • Patient tracking mechanisms and systems are overwhelmed **Tactics:** • Use prerecorded messaging to filter calls that require direct emergency medical dispatch staff contact • Maximize frequent use of emergency broadcast system and media outlets • Implement call triage models to target highest priority calls for response	**Indicators:** • Stabilization or decrease in calls to emergency medical dispatch • Stabilization or decrease in calls to medical advice hotlines • Communication systems, networks, and physical infrastructure returning to baseline functional state **Triggers:** • The number of requests to emergency medical dispatch and for EMS are returning to baseline levels **Tactics:** • Continue to provide the community with information regarding the status of the event • Continue to educate and encourage the community to engage in mitigation measures • Revise dispatch and transport protocols to normalize operations
Staff ***(Refer also to the worker functional capacity table in Toolkit Part 1 [Table 3-1])***	**Indicators:** • Members of the EMD and EMS workforce unable to report for duty due to impassable roads, incapacitated personal vehicles, or other direct effects • Members of the EMD and EMS workforce within the at-risk population for influenza • Members of the EMD and EMS workforce unable to report for duty due to illness, injury, or physical entrapment in residences	**Indicators:** • Overwhelming number of patient with insufficient staff to meet the demand for triage, treatment, and transport • Significant portion of the emergency medical dispatch and EMS workforce is sustaining physical fatigue due to extended work shifts and incident stress • Significant number of the EMD and EMS workforce are affected as disaster victims or incapacitated by the disaster and are unavailable to respond	**Indicators:** • Approaching normal baseline levels of staffing. • Return to normal shift level and staffing • Some emergency medical dispatch and EMS personnel may elect to remain off duty due to family obligations **Triggers:** • The number of emergency medical dispatch and EMS personnel reporting for duty is starting to stabilize • Recovery of EMS personnel from illness and/or injury

Triggers:
- EMS crews are at or approaching minimal staffing
- Loss of 10% or more of the workforce

Tactics:
- Use mutual aid staffing resources
- Prioritize dispatch calls according to potential threat to life, placing non-life threatening calls on a pending status (requires medically trained emergency medical dispatch)
- Reduce staffing requirement from two advanced life support (ALS) providers to one ALS and one basic life support (BLS) provider
- Change ambulance assignments according to closest available units instead of BLS/ALS capability
- Activate non-EMS dispatch protocols in emergency medical dispatch centers and advise patients with minor injuries or illnesses to use their own transportation
- Activate non-transport protocols and disaster triage guidelines for EMS agencies
- Use 211 nurse call centers for triage
- Respond to critical or urgent calls followed by batched transport of stable patients to health care facilities
- Encourage mitigation measures, e.g., mass vaccination, within EMD and EMS workforce
- Transport essential EMS and emergency medical dispatch workers to the workplace via National Guard or other agency
- Provide support to families of EMS and emergency medical dispatch personnel to facilitate the maintenance of the workforce
- Change shift length

- EMS and medical personnel are becoming victims of criminal activity by individuals seeking medications, medical supplies, vaccinations, and expedited treatment or transport

Crisis Triggers:
- Unable to maintain staffing for EMS units
- Staff overwhelmed by number of patients who need care
- Mutual aid staffing resources have been exhausted

Tactics:
- Direct emergency medical dispatch to decline response to calls without evidence of threat to life (requires medically trained EMD)
- Mandatory use of disaster triage guidelines
- Direct EMS to decline transport of assessed patients without significant injury or illness (upon guidance from EMS medical direction)
- Limit resuscitation attempts to witnessed cardiac arrests
- Reduce staffing for ambulances to one EMS provider (upon guidance from EMS medical direction)
- Request additional EMS units through the local emergency operations center (EOC)
- Use public and private mass transportation resources for patients with minor injuries or illnesses
- Integrate transportation resources from out of state and through the Emergency Management Assistance Compact or National Disaster Medical System
- Secure federal, state, regional, and local EMS staffing resources and non-EMS staffing resources (e.g., National Guard)
- Provide appropriate security for EMS crews

Tactics:
- Direct emergency medical dispatch to use initial automated answering systems during spikes of high call volume for medical emergencies, but revert to answering all calls when able
- Initiate a gradual return to normal triage, patient treatment, and transport guidelines
- Initiate a gradual transition to normal staffing levels, work shifts, and sleep cycles
- Initiate plan for reduction and relief of mutual aid resources
- Continue to encourage or require mitigation measures (personal protective equipment [PPE], hand washing, vaccination, etc.)
- Encourage timely engagement in stress management and personal resilience resources

continued

TABLE 7-1
Continued

Indicator Category	Contingency	Crisis	Return Toward Conventional
Space/infrastructure	**Indicators:** • Evacuation routes are becoming crowded • The general public is unable to access timely care in clinics or emergency department • Multiple emergency department and emergency care centers are going on diversion due to overwhelmed capacity • Roads and bridges have collapsed or become structurally unstable **Triggers:** • More than 20-30% of the emergency departments, emergency care centers, and public health clinics have requested additional medical staff or are on diversion • There is a trend within the general public electing not to comply with emergency declaration mitigation directives (e.g., shelter in place, evacuation, driving restrictions) **Tactics:** • Activate and open all alternative care sites, and support these with EMS resources as possible • Activate alternate transport destination and non-transport protocols for emergency medical dispatch and EMS personnel • Encourage the general public to comply with emergency declaration directives, engaging law enforcement assistance if necessary	**Indicators:** • Overwhelming number of patients exceeds the ambulances available • Transport destinations are overwhelmed and do not have the capacity to accept additional patients • Law enforcement resources are overwhelmed or limited • Evacuation routes are no longer passable • The virulence of a biologic agent has increased compared to prior projections • Structural damage to the physical plant of emergency medical dispatch, EMS, or EOC that hampers or incapacitates their operational status • Structural damage to the physical plant of health care facilities that hampers or incapacitates their operational status • Air ambulances are grounded due to weather **Crisis Triggers:** • No available ground ambulances for transport • Mutual aid for additional vehicles is exhausted **Tactics:** • Establish casualty collection points • Use treat and release protocols • Universal use of non-EMS dispatch and non-transport protocols • Use mass transport vehicles (e.g., buses) to transport patients with minor injuries • Use disaster triage guidelines • Designate ambulance transport solely for moderately/seriously ill or injured patients • Use alternative vehicles (e.g., aircraft if weather conditions permit, all terrain vehicles, motorcycles, bicycles, watercraft) to access moderately or severely ill or injured patients when routes of travel that are conducive to ambulances are no longer passable	**Indicators:** • The demand for available ambulances with patient need is better aligned • Roadways are beginning to have reduced volume • Emergency departments and emergency care centers are beginning to accept patients • Structural damage to transport destinations is no longer affecting operational status **Triggers:** • A reduction in health care facilities that are on diversion • Reliable routes of transport have been established for emergency and public safety vehicles **Tactics:** • Continue operational support of alternate transport sites until emergency department and emergency care center report improved flow of inpatients and outpatients • Initiate a gradual transition to conventional transport destinations

Supplies

Indicators:
- EMS agencies report increased use of PPE, medical supplies, medications, or airway management equipment
- Manufacturers of PPE, medical supplies, vaccines, medications, or ventilators report decreased stock available
- Fuel shortages reported

Triggers:
- The available PPE is less than what is needed for the EMS workforce
- The use of medical supplies, medications, vaccines, and antidotes begins to exceed their replacement

Tactics:
- Conservation of PPE
- Conservation of supplies
- Provide medications and vaccinations to designated at-risk populations
- Determine alternate vendors and sources of supplies

Indicators:
- EMS reports inadequate or depleted supply of PPE, medical supplies, medications, or airway management equipment
- Manufacturers of PPE, medical supplies, vaccines, medications, or ventilators report insufficient or depleted stock
- Manufacturers of disaster supplies and recovery equipment report factory closures and/or halted production due to loss of workforce

Crisis Triggers:
- PPE is no longer available
- Vaccinations, medications, or antidotes are depleted to the point that equivalent treatment cannot be provided
- Hospitals can no longer provide supplies or medications to restock ambulances

Tactics:
- Activate crisis standards of care prehospital patient care protocols
- Secure federal, state, regional, and local emergency response assets

Indicators:
- Demand for PPE for EMS personnel is subsiding
- Demand for medical supplies or airway management equipment is reduced
- Manufacturers of PPE, medical supplies, medications, or airway management equipment report improving product availability

Triggers:
- Incident command is receiving reduced requests for additional PPE and medical supplies from EMS personnel
- Emergency departments, emergency care facilities, and hospitals have reduced requests for medications, antidotes, vaccinations, and ventilators
- Manufacturers of disaster supplies and recovery equipment report a return to production

Tactics:
- Assess the current status of the supplies of medications, medical equipment, and PPE
- Request a limited volume of PPE and supplies to prepare for a potential resurgence and to begin replenishing the normal stock of supplies
- Adjust supply allocation guidance toward normal

Decision-Support Tool: Blank Table to Be Completed

Prompted by discussion of the key questions above, participants should fill out this blank table (or multiple tables for different scenarios) with key system indicators and triggers that will drive actions in their own organizations, agencies, and jurisdictions.[4]

Reminders:

- *Indicators* are measures or predictors of changes in demand and/or resource availability; *triggers* are decision points.
- The key questions were designed to facilitate discussion—customized for EMS—about the following four steps to consider when developing indicators and triggers for a specific organization/agency/jurisdiction: (1) identify key response strategies and actions, (2) identify and examine potential indicators, (3) determine trigger points, and (4) determine tactics.
- Discussions about triggers should include (a) triggers for which a "bright line" can be described, and (b) *how* expert decisions to implement tactics would be made using one or more indicators for which no bright line exists. Discussions should consider the benefits of *anticipating* the implementation of tactics, and of *leaning forward* to implement certain tactics in advance of a bright line or when no such line exists.
- The example table may be consulted to promote discussion and to provide a sense of the level of detail and concreteness that is needed to develop useful indicators and triggers for a specific organization/agency/jurisdiction.
- This table is intended to frame discussions and create awareness of information, policy sources, and issues at the agency level to share with other stakeholders. Areas of uncertainty should be noted and clarified with partners.
- Refer back to the toolkit introduction (Chapter 3) for key definitions and concepts.

---

[4] The blank table for participants to complete can be downloaded from the project's website: www.iom.edu/crisisstandards.

Scope and Event Type: _____

Indicator Category	Contingency	Crisis	Return Toward Conventional
Surveillance data	Indicators: Triggers: Tactics:	Indicators: Crisis triggers: Tactics:	Indicators: Triggers: Tactics:
Communications and community infrastructure	Indicators: Triggers: Tactics:	Indicators: Crisis triggers: Tactics:	Indicators: Triggers: Tactics:
Staff	Indicators: Triggers: Tactics:	Indicators: Crisis triggers: Tactics:	Indicators: Triggers: Tactics:
Space/infrastructure	Indicators: Triggers: Tactics:	Indicators: Crisis triggers: Tactics:	Indicators: Triggers: Tactics:
Supplies	Indicators: Triggers: Tactics:	Indicators: Crisis triggers: Tactics:	Indicators: Triggers: Tactics:
Other categories	Indicators: Triggers: Tactics:	Indicators: Crisis triggers: Tactics:	Indicators: Triggers: Tactics:

REFERENCE

IOM (Institute of Medicine). 2012. *Crisis standards of care: A systems framework for catastrophic disaster response.* Washington, DC: The National Academies Press. http://www.nap.edu/openbook.php?record_id=13351 (accessed April 3, 2013).

8: Toolkit Part 2: Hospital and Acute Care

INTRODUCTION

This chapter presents a discussion and decision-support tool to facilitate the development of indicators and triggers that help guide hospital and acute care decision making during a disaster. Because integrated planning across the emergency response system is critical for a coordinated response, it is important to first read the introduction to the toolkit and materials relevant to the entire emergency response system in Chapter 3. It would be helpful to also review the toolkit chapters focused on other stakeholders.

Roles and Responsibilities

Hospitals should ensure they are able to fulfill their mission to provide emergency care and inpatient/outpatient care to all members of the community, including specialty populations they may not normally serve (e.g., burn, trauma, pediatric) through development of response plans to include:

- Incident management systems such as the Hospital Incident Command System (HICS) that are compatible with the National Incident Management System (NIMS);
- Response communication and coordination capabilities with key stakeholders, including other health care organizations in the area, established health care coalitions, emergency management, emergency medical services (EMS), and public health;
- Appropriate space, staff, and supply planning to ensure the ability to meet the needs of a disaster relative to their Hazard Vulnerability Analysis (HVA) and role in the community; and
- Specific planning for scarce resource situations, including the role of incident management, how subject matter experts and/or a clinical care committee[1] are used, triage processes, and the integration with scarce resource management processes at the coalition and jurisdictional levels.

---

[1] "Composed of clinical and administrative leaders at a health care institution, this committee is responsible for prioritizing the allocation of critical life-sustaining interventions. The clinical care committee may also be formed at the health care coalition level (e.g., hospital, primary care, emergency medical services agency, public health, emergency management, and others), playing the role of the disaster medical advisory committee at the regional level. . . . May appoint a triage team . . . to evaluate case-by-case decisions" (IOM, 2012, p. 7-1). See IOM (2012) for additional information about the roles and composition of the clinical care committee and other entities involved in planning and implementing crisis standards of care.

Additional discussion about the roles and responsibilities of hospital and acute care facilities in planning for and implementing crisis standards of care (CSC) is available in the Institute of Medicine's (IOM's) 2012 report *Crisis Standards of Care: A Systems Framework for Catastrophic Disaster Response*. This report also includes planning and implementation templates that outline core functions and tasks.

Key Issues for Hospitals

This brief overview is supported by a more robust discussion of indicators and triggers in the overview chapters as well as by discussion of crisis care planning, strategies, and tactics in the IOM 2012 report and other publications (see Chapter 1).

Hospitals should ensure that they have accounted for the following in their planning for disaster response, and for scarce resource situations in particular:

1. Situational awareness, including information availability and analysis
2. Disaster plan trigger(s)
3. Crisis care trigger(s)

Situational awareness, including information availability and analysis, requires that the hospital can receive, verify when possible, and communicate the information available. This includes understanding sources, formats, availability, and processes for information access, assessment, and action within the facility (e.g., who receives health alerts and what they do with them). The hospital should determine whether it has daily management goals (prediction of discharge date, bed management) where information that may be critical to successful disaster response can be captured to improve efficiency and preparedness concurrently. It may be helpful to brainstorm a list of information and data that would be helpful in making decisions and determine how easy it is to obtain those data, how accurate and useful they will be, and whether or not they are actionable: that is, can the facility take actions to change the variable or not?—an example is bed availability—and what are the likely actions to be taken? Considering information in the facility and regional HVA may be helpful. This will naturally lead to discussions about thresholds and decision making, and potentially to defining facility triggers.

Disaster plan triggers cause activation of the facility emergency operations plan, marking the transition to contingency care. The roles authorized to activate the plan should be able to analyze situational information in order to make this decision. There is often uncertainty, and full plan activation involves significant time and financial impact for the facility. The larger the event, the less uncertainty there may be. Suggested triggers (number of victims by time of day, types of victims) should be available to the decision makers, who should also have the experience to consider the current facility status, the likely impact, and other factors when deciding whether or not to activate. Emergency actions at the unit level can be based on more certain triggers (in case of fire on a unit, perform the following actions), but at the institutional level, many triggers require at least a degree of interpretation of the situation (e.g., complete vs. partial hospital evacuation, destination of evacuated psychiatric inpatients) that is not amenable to binary criteria.

Crisis care triggers should shift the incident management perspective to consideration of the overall, rather than individual patient demand and should prompt

- Use of adaptive strategies to reduce impact—extension of substitute, conserve, adapt, and reuse strategies, and introduction of reallocation if required;
- Creation of a clinical care committee (or at minimum, involvement of subject matter experts) to provide recommendations;
- Analysis of impact (using specific indicators for the resources in shortage) and development of recommended strategies and tactics to cope with the deficit;
- Proactive strategies to acquire additional resources from coalition or emergency management partners, or manage those available in a congruent fashion;
- Communication to staff, patients, and families about the situation and what is being done in concert with hospital and community (Joint Information System) incident management; and
- Determination if legal or regulatory actions are required to support crisis care strategies (e.g., from emergency management, public health).

Crisis situations may begin with a discrete indicator of excess demand (e.g., inadequate numbers of ventilators, medications, or staff), which triggers activation of the crisis care process, but does not necessarily result in allocation or triage *decisions*, which are the last resort in crisis care (e.g., anesthesia machines may be used, substitute medications found, or staffing patterns changed to avoid triage). Optimally, this planning process begins before the trigger threshold is reached, as the shortage was anticipated based on monitoring of indicators (e.g., examining pandemic epidemiology vs. supplies). Sometimes, crisis situations may develop without notice, and staff in these situations should have guidelines to follow both from an operations (adaptive strategies for space, staff, etc.) and an ethical (triage decisions) perspective. Facilities should determine *what* specifically occurs and *who* becomes involved when the incident commander activates the crisis care annex to the emergency operations plan. This should involve discrete triggers as well as the option to consider other factors and initiate the crisis care plan proactively based on indicators of demand. Factors other than shortage of clinical care resources may contribute to a crisis situation, including the demands of providing information and support for families seeking loved ones, family members of patients, and mass fatality situations.

Of critical importance is emphasizing the interdependency of the health care response system among hospitals, EMS, other health care facilities (including the outpatient sector), and effective interventions and risk communication coordinated by public health and emergency management. Planning with these entities to ensure an integrated response with joint objective and strategy setting is critical. Discussions based on the discipline-specific templates may be helpful to frame common issues and key interfaces/areas of need.

DISCUSSION AND DECISION-SUPPORT TOOL

Suggested participants for a discussion focused on hospital and acute care are listed below. Building on the scenarios and overarching key questions presented in Chapter 3, this tool contains additional questions to help participants drill down on the key issues and details for hospital and acute care. It also contains a table that provides example hospital and acute care indicators, triggers, and tactics, and a blank chart for participants to complete. The scenarios, questions, and example chart are intended to provoke discussion that will help participants fill in the blank chart for their own situation.[2] Participants may choose to complete a single, general blank chart, or one each for various scenarios from their HVA.

Discussion Participants

Suggested participants for a discussion focused on hospitals and acute care facilities are listed below.

- Hospital administration;
- Hospital emergency management;
- Chief medical officer;
- Legal counsel;
- Subject matter experts (e.g., infection control for the pandemic scenario or trauma program manager for the earthquake scenario); and
- Health care coalition members.

Following these initial discussions, sharing and coordination of this information with a much broader range of stakeholders (e.g., blood bank, EMS, trauma networks, community Department of Defense medical liaisons, federally qualified health centers, nursing homes, public health, primary care providers and emergency management, elected officials, and others listed in part one of the toolkit) is critical to an integrated response.

Key Questions: Slow-Onset Scenario

The questions below are focused on the slow-onset influenza pandemic scenario presented in Chapter 3[3]:

1. What potential indicator data are available at the community or state level and who coordinates or has access to these (systems data, epidemiologic data, alerts)?
4. Who monitors and interprets these data; how are they communicated or used in decision making?
5. What additional information could be accessed during an incident or event that would be helpful to guide facility/agency actions?
6. Do any defined actions or notifications occur once an indicator is noted or a threshold exceeded?
7. Is the facility an active participant in their regional health care coalition and if so, what resources are available, what is the trigger for requesting them, and how are they requested (medical coordination center)?
8. What are the crisis care triggers for the institution that would signify a need to implement CSC? Are these similar to other hospitals within the health care coalition?

---

[2] The blank table for participants to complete can be downloaded from the project's website: www.iom.edu/crisisstandards.

[3] These questions are provided to help start discussion; additional important questions may arise during the course of discussion. The questions are aimed at raising issues related to indicators and triggers, and are not comprehensive of all important questions related to disaster preparedness and response.

9. At what threshold (indicator or trigger) does interfacility communication and/or coordination begin (including EMS, emergency management, public health, and coalition/community health care organizations)?

10. How do the facility and coalition share information (including impact, resource availability, case and clinical information) with state and local public health agencies to optimize situational awareness and resource management?

11. What triggers exist at the state level to provide declarations of emergency (and/or regulatory and liability protections) from public health or emergency management? If there are not predesignated triggers, how are requests handled on these actions?

12. How does the institution internally and externally (with local public health) recognize the need for and support alternate care sites?

Key Questions: No-Notice Scenario

The questions below are focused on the no-notice earthquake scenario presented in Chapter 3:

1. What alerts, system information, or situation information does the facility receive from outside agencies and how is it (or are they) processed?

2. What internal information is available from which indicator and trigger thresholds may be derived (e.g., information technology system status, staffing, bed capacity, ventilator availability, operating room use, supplies)?

3. What additional information would be needed during an event to inform decisions on level of care that can be provided?

4. What are thresholds that can reasonably be set for review or action based on specific external or internal measures (i.e., how is the information converted to staff actions, such as activating the disaster plan or calling back select staff)?

5. How does the facility determine staff absences, illness rates, availability to report, and other data that may be critical for response?

6. What information is available or potentially available to serve as a facility "dashboard" to monitor system status? How does this system reflect disaster status? (e.g., use of additional beds, use of procedure area beds for patient care)?

7. When a no-notice event moves immediately to a crisis trigger threshold, what specific actions are defined for staff to implement—not only incident management systems but also triage processes and policies?

8. How is support provided to providers and their families to allow them to reduce stress and focus on their job duties?

9. How would decisions be made about facility evacuation or shelter-in-place (e.g., decision tools, policy, damage assessment tools)? How are these decisions communicated to the licensing or regulatory agencies?

10. What resources exist within the regional coalition/regional trauma network for impacted hospitals (e.g., diversion, specific staff, or supply resources)?

11. Are any specific indicators and triggers needed for specialty care (e.g., burn, trauma, pediatrics) or other at-risk individuals?

Decision-Support Tool: Example Table

The indicators, triggers, and tactics shown in Table 8-1 are examples to help promote discussion and provide a sense of the level of detail and concreteness that is needed to develop useful indicators and triggers for a specific organization/agency/jurisdiction; they are not intended to be exhaustive or universally applicable. Prompted by discussion of the key questions above, discussion participants should fill out a blank table, focusing on key system indicators and triggers that will drive actions in their own organizations, agencies, and jurisdictions. As a reminder, *indicators* are measures or predictors of changes in demand and/or resource availability; *triggers* are decision points (refer back to the toolkit introduction [Chapter 3] for key definitions and concepts).

The example triggers shown in the table mainly are ones in which a "bright line" distinguishes functionally different levels of care (conventional, contingency, crisis). Because of the nature of this type of trigger, they can be described more concretely and can be included in a bulleted list. It is important to recognize, however, that expert analysis of one or more indicators may also trigger implementation of key response plans, actions, and tactics. This may be particularly true in a slow-onset scenario. In all cases, but particularly in the absence of bright lines, decisions may need to be made to *anticipate* upcoming problems and the implementation of tactics and to *lean forward* by implementing certain tactics before reaching the bright line or when no such line exists. These decision points vary according to the situation and are based on analysis of multiple inputs, recommendations, and, in certain circumstances, previous experience. Discussions about these tables should cover *how* such decisions would be made, even if the specifics cannot be included in a bulleted list in advance. Note that these sample indicators, triggers, and tactics are geared toward a smaller community hospital and are not comprehensive in scope, but meant to support discussion at the facility level.

TABLE 8-1
Example Hospital Indicators, Triggers, and Tactics for Transitions Along the Continuum of Care

Indicator Category	Contingency	Crisis	Return Toward Conventional
Community and communications infrastructure	**Indicators:** • Impact on community, including transportation and communications infrastructure **Triggers:** • Loss of paging and/or cellular service in area • Loss of phone service to hospital • Loss of electrical service to hospital • Closure of transit system **Tactics:** • Use alternate communications strategies such as mass media and text messages, 700 or 800 MHz radio, satellite phones, HAM radios • Provide employee alternate transportation options and on-site temporary housing • Provide information to staff, visitors, and family members about impacts and response actions/options	**Indicators:** • Community-wide and likely prolonged impact on infrastructure affecting employee homes, transportation, and communication **Crisis Triggers:** • Loss of electrical power or generator failure **Tactics:** • Hospital evacuation/diversion if possible • Consider whether shelter-in-place is an option • Provide bag-valve ventilation for ventilator-dependent patients or place on battery-operated transport ventilators • Anticipate need to switch to gravity drip IV medications with monitoring of drip rates as pump batteries fail	**Indicators:** • Restoration of services and transportation access **Triggers:** • Restored electrical service **Tactics:** • Scale back tactics or revert to conventional operations
Surveillance data	**Indicators:** • Pandemic or epidemic (e.g., SARS) virus detected • Health alert or other notification received • Natural disaster occurs or mass casualty incident (MCI) declaration in community • Epidemiologic forecasts (Centers for Disease Control and Prevention [CDC], etc.) • Local surveillance/epidemiology data • Standard metrics such as NEDOCS (National Emergency Department Overcrowding Score) • Regional/community emergency department (ED) volume, ED wait times/boarding times • Regional/community hospital capacity or subset data, such as available intensive care unit (ICU) beds	**Indicators:** • Epidemiologic projections will exceed resources available **Crisis Triggers:** • Epidemiology projections exceed surge capacity of facility for space or specific capability (e.g., critical care)—see below space and supply considerations, as triggers should be based on depletion of available resources	**Indicators:** • Surveillance streams show decline in activity • Improvement in regional/community ED volumes/wait times/boarding times **Triggers:** • Not specified for predictive data, will adjust based on specific actionable data **Tactics:** • Stand down incident management (scaled) • Lengthen duration of planning cycles • Reduce/deactivate regional information exchange • Facility practices revert toward conventional • Revert to normal system monitoring (defer this until incident clearly concludes)

continued

TABLE 8-1
Continued

Indicator Category	Contingency	Crisis	Return Toward Conventional
Surveillance data (continued)	**Triggers:** • Receipt of health alert triggers group notification by receiving infection prevention personnel • Disaster plan activated when >X seriously injured victims expected at facility—Hospital Command Center opens • "Full capacity" plan initiated when ED wait times exceed X hours **Tactics:** • Change or increase monitoring parameters, additional situational awareness activities • Partial or full activation of incident command system/hospital command center • Communication/coordination with stakeholders/coalition partners • Change hours, staffing, internal processes in accord with facility plans • Assess predicted impact on institution		
Staff *[Refer also to the worker functional capacity table in Toolkit Part 1 (Table 3-1)]*	**Indicators:** • Increasing staff absenteeism • Specialized staff needed (pediatrics, burn, geriatrics) for incident patients • School closures • Staff work action anticipated (e.g., strike) • High patient census • Staffing hours adjustment required to maintain coverage • Staffing supervision model changes required to maintain coverage **Triggers:** • X% staff ill call rate prompts notification of emergency management group • School closures across area trigger opening of staff day care • Normal staff to patient ratios exceeded • Specific staff expertise demands exceeded (e.g., mass burn event—depletion of burn nurses)	**Indicators:** • Increasing staff requirements in face of increasing demand • Contingency spaces maximized • Contingency staffing maximized **Crisis Triggers:** • Unable to safely increase staff to patient ratios or broaden supervisory responsibilities • Lack of qualified staff for specific cares—especially those with high life-safety impact **Tactics:** • Tailor responsibilities to expertise, diverting nontechnical or non-essential care to others • Recruit and credential staff from volunteer (Medical Reserve Corps [MRC], Emergency System for Advance Registration of Volunteer Health Professionals [ESAR-VHP]) or federal sources (Disaster Medical Assistance Team [DMAT], other National Disaster Medical System [NDMS] source, etc.)	**Indicators:** • Staff impact is reduced, schools back in session, damage to community mitigated • Staff absenteeism reduced • Specialty staff obtained or demand decreased **Trigger:** • Staff to patient ratios of 1:X achieved on medical floor **Tactics:** • Shorten shift lengths • Adjust staff to patient ratios toward normal • Transition toward usual staff—releasing less qualified staff first • Resume care routines • Resume administrative duties

Tactics:
- Assess likely impact on facility
- Hold staff
- Change hours, staffing patterns
- Change staff to patient ratios
- Specialty staff provide only specialty/technical care, while other staff provide more general care
- Callback, obtain equivalent staff from coalition, hiring, administrative staff
- Change charting responsibilities
- Curtail nonessential staffing (cancel elective cases, specialty clinic visits, etc.)
- Provide support for staff (and their families as required) to help them continue to work and provide quality care (e.g., stress "immunization," rest periods, housing support)

- Establish remote consultation of specialized services such as telemedicine, phone triage, etc., if possible
- Evacuate patients to other facilities with appropriate staff available

Space/ infrastructure			
Indicators: - Increased ED volumes - Increased clinic/outpatient volumes - Increased inpatient census - Increased pending admits/ED boarding **Triggers:** - Inpatient census exceeds conventional beds - Damage to infrastructure - Clinics unable to accommodate demand for acute care - >X hours ED boarding time - Electronic health record downtime - Telephone or Internet systems failures **Tactics:** - Expand hours of outpatient care - Open additional outpatient care space by adjusting specialty clinic space/times - Provide "inpatient" care on preinduction, postanesthesia care, other equivalent areas - Divert patients to clinics/other facilities - Transfer patients to other facilities - "Reverse triage" appropriate patients home (with appropriate home care) - Implement downtime procedures for IT systems	**Indicators:** - Inpatient/outpatient contingency spaces maximized or near-maximized - Escalating or sustained demand on ED/outpatient despite implementing contingency strategies - Damage to infrastructure affecting critical systems **Crisis Triggers:** - Contingency inpatient beds maximized (may include subset of ICU, burn, pediatrics, etc.) - Contingency outpatient adaptations inadequate to meet demand using equivalent spaces or strategies - Damage to infrastructure affecting critical systems *and* presenting a safety issue to staff/patients **Tactics:** - Establish nontraditional alternate care locations (e.g., auditorium, tents, conference rooms), recognizing governmental role in authorizing waivers - "Reverse triage" stable patients to these areas, move stable ICU patients to monitored bed areas (i.e., step-down units deliver ICU-level care)	**Indicators:** - Favorable epidemiologic curves - Restoration of critical system function - ED/outpatient volumes decreasing **Trigger:** - Patients able to be matched to appropriate areas for care **Tactics:** - Transitional movement of sickest patients back into ICU environment - Broaden admission criteria - Reduce/eliminate care in nontraditional spaces (stop providing assessment/care in non-patient care areas/cot-based) - Shift toward normal hours	

continued

TABLE 8-1
Continued

Indicator Category	Contingency	Crisis	Return Toward Conventional
Space/ infrastructure (continued)		• Consider other methods of outpatient care, including telephone treatment and prescribing • Change admission criteria—manage as outpatients with support/early follow-up • Evacuate patients to other facilities in the region/state/nation that have appropriate capabilities and capacity	
Supplies	**Indicators:** • Vendor supply or delivery disruption • Supply consumption/use rates • Epidemiology of event predicts supply impact **Triggers:** • Event epidemiology predicts ventilator or other specific resource shortages (e.g., pediatric equipment) • Medication/vaccine supply limited • Consumption rates of personal protective equipment (PPE) unsustainable • Vendor shortages impact ability to provide normal resources **Tactics:** • Use nontraditional vendors • Obtain from coalition facilities/ stockpiles (including potential state/ federal sources) • Conserve, substitute, or adapt functionally equivalent resources; reuse if appropriate	**Indicators:** • Coalition lack of available ventilators • Anesthesia machines and other adaptive ventilation strategies in use • Coalition/vendor lack of available critical supplies/medications **Crisis Triggers:** • Inadequate ventilators (or other life-sustaining technology) for all patients that require them • Inadequate supplies of medications or supplies that cannot be effectively conserved or substituted for without risk of disability or death without treatment **Tactics:** • Implement triage team/clinical care committee process • Determine bridging therapies (bag-valve ventilation, etc.) • Coordinate care/triage policies with coalition facilities (in no-notice event, this may not be possible) • Triage access to live-saving resources (ventilators, blood products, specific medications) and reallocate as required to meet demand according to state/ regional consensus recommendations • Restrict medications to select indications • Restrict PPE to high-risk exposures (and/or permit PPE reuse) • Reuse or reallocate resources when possible (benefit should outweigh risks of reuse; reallocate only when no alternatives—see criteria in IOM, 2012)	**Indicators:** • Reduced use of PPE or other supplies • Reduced caseload or demand for care and services • Improved delivery of supplies • Reduced need for ventilator or other triage **Triggers:** • Able to provide contingency ventilation and critical care strategies to all that require them **Tactics:** • Retriage patients as resources become available • Broaden indications for interventions as conditions improve • Transition back from reallocation and reuse to safer adaptive and conservation strategies • Loosen restrictions on use of supplies

Decision-Support Tool: Blank Table to Be Completed

Prompted by discussion of the key questions above, participants should fill out this blank table (or multiple tables for different scenarios) with key system indicators and triggers that will drive actions in their own organizations, agencies, and jurisdictions.[4]

Reminders:

- *Indicators* are measures or predictors of changes in demand and/or resource availability; *triggers* are decision points.
- The key questions were designed to facilitate discussion—customized for hospitals and acute care—about the following four steps to consider when developing indicators and triggers for a specific organization/agency/jurisdiction: (1) identify key response strategies and actions, (2) identify and examine potential indicators, (3) determine trigger points, (4) determine tactics.
- Discussions about triggers should include (a) triggers for which a "bright line" can be described, and (b) *how* expert decisions to implement tactics would be made using one or more indicators for which no bright line exists. Discussions should consider the benefits of *anticipating* the implementation of tactics, and of *leaning forward* to implement certain tactics in advance of a bright line or when no such line exists.
- The example table may be consulted to promote discussion and to provide a sense of the level of detail and concreteness that is needed to develop useful indicators and triggers for a specific organization/agency/jurisdiction.
- This table is intended to frame discussions and create awareness of information, policy sources, and issues at the agency level to share with other stakeholders. Areas of uncertainty should be noted and clarified with partners.
- Refer back to the toolkit introduction (Chapter 3) for key definitions and concepts.

---

[4] The blank table for participants to complete can be downloaded from the project's website: www.iom.edu/crisisstandards.

Scope and Event Type: _____

Indicator Category	Contingency	Crisis	Return Toward Conventional
Surveillance data	Indicators: Triggers: Tactics:	Indicators: Crisis triggers: Tactics:	Indicators: Triggers: Tactics:
Communications and community infrastructure	Indicators: Triggers: Tactics:	Indicators: Crisis triggers: Tactics:	Indicators: Triggers: Tactics:
Staff	Indicators: Triggers: Tactics:	Indicators: Crisis triggers: Tactics:	Indicators: Triggers: Tactics:
Space/infrastructure	Indicators: Triggers: Tactics:	Indicators: Crisis triggers: Tactics:	Indicators: Triggers: Tactics:
Supplies	Indicators: Triggers: Tactics:	Indicators: Crisis triggers: Tactics:	Indicators: Triggers: Tactics:
Other categories	Indicators: Triggers: Tactics:	Indicators: Crisis triggers: Tactics:	Indicators: Triggers: Tactics:

REFERENCE

IOM (Institute of Medicine). 2012. *Crisis standards of care: A systems framework for catastrophic disaster response.* Washington, DC: The National Academies Press. http://www.nap.edu/openbook.php?record_id=13351 (accessed April 3, 2013).

9: Toolkit Part 2: Out-of-Hospital Care

INTRODUCTION

This chapter presents a discussion and decision-support tool to facilitate the development of indicators and triggers that help guide out-of-hospital care decision making during a disaster. Because integrated planning across the emergency response system is critical for a coordinated response, it is important to first read the introduction to the toolkit and materials relevant to the entire emergency response system in Chapter 3. Review the toolkit chapters focused on other stakeholders also would be helpful.

Roles and Responsibilities

The out-of-hospital care delivery system is very diverse, with many roles and responsibilities within a community. These include community-based health care provided in diverse ambulatory care environments (public, private, tribal, veterans health, military), home health and hospice, assisted living and skilled nursing, specialty care and resources, and others. Additional discussion about the roles and responsibilities of out-of-hospital and alternate care systems in planning for and implementing crisis standards of care is available in the Institute of Medicine's (IOM's) 2012 report *Crisis Standards of Care: A Systems Framework for Catastrophic Disaster Response*. This report also includes planning and implementation templates that outline core functions and tasks.

Planning and coordination among these entities can be difficult because no single entity has jurisdiction. The components of this broad care system need to work together to engage in disaster planning activities to maximize resources and ensure that the needs of patients, clients, and residents are met. In the large majority of situations, the out-of-hospital providers need to work collaboratively with the other emergency response sectors because it is a component of a larger system of health care resources. For example, hospitals and local agencies may need to work together to ensure that patients can be discharged safely to their homes, including assessing whether the home was damaged and determining whether basic food, water, and heating needs are sufficient. It is evident that the majority of health care services are provided in the outpatient setting, highlighting the importance of these specialized care providers in disaster response. In certain circumstances, ambulatory care should make linkages to the professional associations that oversee the policy formulation for a number of population-specific entities (e.g., renal response, long-term care, palliative care).

Key Issues

The out-of-hospital system could be impacted directly by the crisis scenario (e.g., damage to a long-term care facility or dialysis center) or indirectly by requested support for surge in the other components of the health care spectrum (e.g., early discharge from hospitals creating surge in home care needs). The engagement of the out-of-hospital care delivery partners with local public health and in health care coalitions is critical to ensuring that resources are maximized during disasters or public health or medical emergencies. Maximization of out-of-hospital care improves access to care (and thus potentially avoids complications) and reduces the pressure on emergency departments and inpatient care. Creating bidirectional communication linkages among the components of the out-of-hospital providers and with the other traditional medical providers helps to ensure the ability to function effectively during crises. This is also important for better coordination with emergency management, which has the primary responsibility for ensuring the continuity of private-sector resources.

DISCUSSION AND DECISION-SUPPORT TOOL

Suggested participants for a discussion focused on out-of-hospital care are listed below. Building on the scenarios and overarching key questions presented in Chapter 3, this tool contains additional questions to help participants drill down on the key issues and details for out-of-hospital care. It also contains a chart that provides example out-of-hospital care indicators, triggers, and tactics, and a blank chart for participants to complete. The scenarios, questions, and example chart are intended to provoke discussion that will help participants fill in the blank chart for their own situation.[1] Participants may choose to complete a single, general blank chart, or one each for various scenarios from their Hazard Vulnerability Analysis.

Discussion Participants

Suggested participants for a discussion focused on out-of-hospital are listed below.

- Local public health;
- Home care agencies;
- Assisted living;
- Long-term care;
- Skilled nursing facilities;
- Outpatient clinics (multispecialty group practices, federally qualified health centers, dialysis centers, etc.);
- Private practice community;
- Hospice care;
- Specialty associations (e.g., dialysis networks);
- Behavioral health providers;
- Poison control and other call centers;

---

[1] The blank table for participants to complete can be downloaded from the project's website: www.iom.edu/crisisstandards.

- Pharmacies; and
- Building facilities managers, especially in urban areas.

Key Questions: Slow-Onset Scenario

The questions below are focused on the slow-onset influenza pandemic scenario presented in Chapter 3[2]:

1. What relevant information is accessible pertaining to out-of-hospital (home care, hospice, long-term care, clinics, etc.) capacity and resources?
2. What additional information could be accessed in pre-event planning for contingency or crisis response?
3. How would this information drive actions?
4. What patient care delivery changes would be implemented, which ones are needed to address the scenario, and when would they be initiated?
5. What patient care delivery assets are preserved (prioritized) in order to support basic health care delivery needs? What information is needed to make the decision to conserve resources?
6. What indicators demonstrate that patient care services can no longer be sustained?
7. What would be done when durable medical equipment providers can no longer provide home oxygen? Does the agency have contingency plans or contracts to augment current resources?
8. What alternate care facility plans have been developed and exercised in the community and what is each stakeholder's role in these plans? Are personnel or a facility available to serve in this capacity for response?
9. What would be done when alternate care facilities are at capacity?
10. What would be done when hospice patients are seeking treatment in acute care facilities?
11. How do stakeholders ensure consistency and coordination of community-derived patient care goals?
12. How does the agency ensure that its communications messages are shared with the Joint Information Center (JIC)?
13. In what ways do community-based care providers interface with the broader public health and medical response community (Emergency Support Function- [ESF-] 8)?
14. How is the interdependence among the organizations within a given medical specialty and with other health care delivery systems managed?
15. What plans are made to ensure mission-critical functionality?
16. Does another care model depend on the facility as part of the development of its surge response plans? If so, how is the delivery of care to patients prioritized?

---

[2] Note: Many of the key questions are intended to ensure that planners are thinking about the situational awareness that they will need to make decisions regarding the transition of care in the outpatient setting along the surge continuum, from conventional to contingency to crisis care response. In many cases, the out-of-hospital care facilities will not necessarily have access to such information on an agency basis. Recognition of community partnerships that may facilitate access to this needed information is an important aspect of planning for such events. In particular, participation in local/regional Healthcare Coalitions (see ASPR, 2012) will be a useful entrée to coordinating out-of-hospital care with the health and medical community. These questions are provided to help start discussion; additional important questions may arise during the course of discussion. The questions are aimed at raising issues related to indicators and triggers, and are not comprehensive of all important questions related to disaster preparedness and response.

17. How does the facility prepare for evacuation due to incapacitation or shelter-in-place if instructed by local emergency management?

Key Questions: No-Notice Scenario

The questions below are focused on the no-notice earthquake scenario presented in Chapter 3:

1. What relevant information is accessible to pertaining to out-of-hospital (home care, hospice, long-term care, clinics, etc.) capacity and resources?
2. How would this information drive actions?
3. What planning efforts have been undertaken to promote resilience and continuity of operations in the face of severe infrastructure damage? Does the agency have redundant mechanisms to communicate with personnel?
4. In the setting of presumed communications infrastructure disruption, are there alternate ways to receive needed situational awareness?
5. How is damage assessment information sent and received within the context of the broad public health and medical response system?
6. What systems or processes are in place to obtain universal damage assessments and how are damage assessments communicated to staff, personnel, patients, families, and vendors?
7. What strategies can be used to prevent home ventilator patients and those seeking medication from needing to go to overtaxed hospitals to seek assistance?
8. What would be done when roads are impassible and vulnerable home care, hospice, and long-term care patients cannot be reached? Are these strategies routinely communicated to patients currently receiving care (alternate dialysis sites, home preparedness kits, etc.)?
9. What would be done when there are not enough staff for those seeking care at alternate care sites?
10. What systems are in place to manage the medical records to preserve key patient information and support continuity of care if evacuation is required?
11. How do stakeholders ensure consistency and coordination of community-derived patient care goals?
12. How does the agency ensure that its communications messages are shared with the JIC?
13. In what ways does the facility/agency interface with the broader public health and medical response community (ESF-8)?
14. How is interdependence among organizations managed within the medical specialty and with other health care delivery systems?
15. What plans are made to ensure mission-critical functionality?
16. Does another care model depend on the facility as part of the development of its surge response plans? If so, how is the delivery of care to patients prioritized?
17. How does the facility prepare for evacuation due to incapacitation or shelter-in-place if instructed by local emergency management?

Decision-Support Tool: Example Table

This example table (Table 9-1) provides *sample* indicators, triggers, and tactics for home care, ambulatory care, long-term care, and skilled nursing facilities. Because of the extensive variability among these types of entities, developing customized indicators and triggers for participants' own situations will be particularly important. The indicators, triggers, and tactics shown in the table are intended to help promote discussion and provide a sense of the level of detail and concreteness that is needed to develop useful indicators and triggers for a specific organization/agency/jurisdiction; they are not intended to be exhaustive or universally applicable. Prompted by discussion of the key questions above, discussion participants should fill out a blank table, focusing on key system indicators and triggers that will drive actions in their own organizations, agencies, and jurisdictions. As a reminder, *indicators* are measures or predictors of changes in demand and/or resource availability; *triggers* are decision points (refer back to the toolkit introduction [Chapter 3] for key definitions and concepts).

The example triggers shown in the table mainly are ones in which a "bright line" distinguishes functionally different levels of care (conventional, contingency, crisis). Because of the nature of this type of trigger, they can be described more concretely and can be included in a bulleted list. It is important to recognize, however, that expert analysis of one or more indicators may also trigger implementation of key response plans, actions, and tactics. This may be particularly true in a slow-onset scenario. In all cases, but particularly in the absence of "bright lines," decisions may need to be made to *anticipate* upcoming problems and the implementation of tactics and to *lean forward* by implementing certain tactics before reaching the bright line or when no such line exists. These decision points vary according to the situation and are based on analysis of multiple inputs, recommendations, and, in certain circumstances, previous experience. Discussions about these tables should cover *how* such decisions would be made, even if the specifics cannot be included in a bulleted list in advance.

TABLE 9-1
Example Out-of-Hospital Indicators, Triggers, and Tactics for Transitions Along the Continuum of Care

Indicator Category	Contingency	Crisis	Return Toward Conventional
Surveillance data	**Indicators:** • Epidemiological surveillance data highlights specific population predilection (e.g., pediatrics, geriatrics) • Local/regional surveillance and epidemiological data **Triggers:** • Increasing discharges from hospital • Increased demand for patient care services **Tactics:** • Coordinate with local/regional health care coalition • Anticipate impact of these events on sustainment of patient care service delivery and make adjustments based on existing emergency operations plans	**Indicators:** • Dramatic demand for patient care services (e.g., surge in hospital discharges) **Crisis Triggers:** • Unable to deliver home care to meet patient needs • Large numbers of long-term care patients requiring hospitalization due to increasing acuity • Failure to adapt to changing conditions, including ability to expand capacity of services **Tactics:** • Postpone elective appointments • Implement changes to patient care service delivery and make adjustments based on existing emergency operations plans	**Indicators:** • Normal patient care census and length of stay at hospitals • Decreasing disease burden based on surveillance/epidemiological data **Triggers:** • Demand for services lessens and/or availability of resources improves **Tactics:** • Patient care delivery adjusted toward baseline
Community and communications infrastructure	**Indicators:** • Communications are delayed because of partial damage to infrastructure • Utility (e.g., power/water) failures impacting patients who depend on technology (e.g., home ventilator and dialysis patients) and/or long-term care and other utility-dependent facilities **Triggers:** • Inability to track patients during mass evacuation with wide geographic dispersal • Sole reliance on paper-based (minimal) patient care records **Tactics:** • Adjust patient charting requirements	**Indicators:** • Communications infrastructure is severely damaged and will take weeks to restore • Surge of technology-dependent patients seeking care at hospitals **Crisis Triggers:** • Absence of patient care records or inability to provide patient care records • Home care and hospice providers unable to make visits, unable to contact clients **Tactics:** • Emergency plans put in place for managing home-bound patients • Establishment of alternate care sites to manage outpatient surge • Use of surge response tactics, including nurse triage lines, expanded scope of practice for pharmacy/emergency medical services	**Indicators:** • Communications are returning to normal • Utility restoration allows technology-dependent patients to return to their usual care **Triggers:** • Evacuated residents returning to long-term care facilities • Home care providers able to contact patients **Tactics:** • Ability to use standard patient care records and reporting mechanisms reestablished

Staff

(Refer also to the worker functional capacity table in Toolkit Part 1 [Table 3-1])

Indicators:
- Decreased availability of staff for work; increasing staff absenteeism
- Closure of schools
- Travel restrictions and/or reduced mass transportation impedes movement of staff to work

Triggers:
- Need for staffing augmentation through Emergency System for Advance Registration of Volunteer Health Professionals (ESAR-VHP) and Medical Reserve Corps (MRC)

Tactics:
- Adjust staffing hours and routines to accommodate more patients
- Consider provisions needed to allow family members to augment care

Indicators:
- Critical shortages of staff in outpatient clinics, home and hospice care, and long-term care facilities
- Out-of-hospital sector staff are being asked to volunteer (e.g., MRC) to provide care to higher acuity patients (e.g., alternate care sites/hospital surge)

Crisis Triggers:
- Unable to provide necessary health care staff to support patient needs (e.g., home care visits less frequent than indicated and change in provider to patient ratios, families of patients and staff seeking care at long-term care facilities)

Tactics:
- Staffing in long-term care facilities predominantly provided by family members
- Coordination of care with neighbors and other community-based assets
- Home care staff designated as emergency responders so they can travel and access gasoline supplies to see critically ill home care patients.

Indicators:
- Staff available for work
- Schools reopen

Triggers:
- Sufficient staff available so family members no longer need to provide care
- Home and hospice personnel are able to make home visits

Tactics:
- Staffing hours and routines return to conventional operations

continued

TABLE 9-1
Continued

Indicator Category	Contingency	Crisis	Return Toward Conventional
Space/infrastructure	**Indicators:** • Increasing mortality due to event • Community-wide sanitation and food service delivery impacted by event • Travel restrictions due to disruption of transportation infrastructure **Triggers:** • Infrastructure loss in community, including loss of utilities (supply of gasoline for travel, electricity, etc.) **Tactics:** • Expand hours of care in existing outpatient setting • Establish shelter care/use alternate care facilities to manage patient care needs Dual purpose out-of-hospital clinics to accept surge (e.g., federally qualified health centers [FQHCs]) • Long-term care facilities and home care accepting early discharges from hospitals	**Indicators:** • Mass fatalities • Critical shortages of sanitation and food • Transportation infrastructure severely disrupted • Need for mass fatality management **Crisis Triggers:** • Many home care and hospice patients calling ambulances requesting transport to hospitals to seek care/admission (no longer able to be managed at home) • Alternate care facilities beyond capacity • FQHCs are damaged and unable to provide surge capacity • Long-term care facilities damaged and destination facilities unable to accept transfers **Tactics:** • Establish federal alternate care sites (e.g., Federal Medical Stations) • Use alternate spaces for management of decedents (e.g., mass fatality plan implementation); engagement of Disaster Mortuary Assistance Teams	**Indicators:** • Decreasing mortality rate so local resources able to manage fatalities • Sanitation and food are no longer in short supply • Alternate transportation methods have been identified and deployed **Triggers:** • Home care and hospice patients able to return home • Remains are processed by local resources • Alternate care facilities are no longer needed • Long-term care facilities and FQHCs returning to normal operations **Tactics:** • Demobilization of federal resources • Closing alternate care facilities • Outpatient clinics return to normal operations
Equipment/supplies	**Indicators:** • Some shortages of critical supplies noted for outpatient clinics, home care, and hospice patients **Triggers:** • Demand for key equipment and supplies exceeds available resources **Tactics:** • Reusing/repurposing key equipment and supplies in order to meet demands	**Indicators:** • Supplies targeted to this sector are diverted to higher acuity patients (e.g., hospital-based patients) • Critical shortages require rationing of supplies • Reusing, repurposing of equipment and supplies no longer meet the needs **Crisis Triggers:** • Difficult decisions required to fairly allocate available resources • Rationing of equipment and supplies **Tactics:** • Centralize supply distribution to support fair allocation of scarce resources (this may require limitation of certain hospital-based services in favor of supporting outpatient management)	**Indicators:** • Increasing supplies are available **Triggers:** • Demand no longer exceeds available resources **Tactics:** • Reestablishing normal supply chains • Centralized equipment distribution discontinued

Decision-Support Tool: Blank Table to Be Completed

Prompted by discussion of the key questions above, participants should fill out this blank table (or multiple tables for different scenarios) with key system indicators and triggers that will drive actions in their own organizations, agencies, and jurisdictions.[3]

Reminders:

- *Indicators* are measures or predictors of changes in demand and/or resource availability; *triggers* are decision points.
- The key questions were designed to facilitate discussion—customized for out-of-hospital care—about the following four steps to consider when developing indicators and triggers for a specific organization/agency/jurisdiction: (1) identify key response strategies and actions, (2) identify and examine potential indicators, (3) determine trigger points, and (4) determine tactics.
- Discussions about triggers should include (a) triggers for which a "bright line" can be described, and (b) *how* expert decisions to implement tactics would be made using one or more indicators for which no bright line exists. Discussions should consider the benefits of *anticipating* the implementation of tactics, and of *leaning forward* to implement certain tactics in advance of a bright line or when no such line exists.
- The example table may be consulted to promote discussion and to provide a sense of the level of detail and concreteness that is needed to develop useful indicators and triggers for a specific organization/agency/jurisdiction.
- This table is intended to frame discussions and create awareness of information, policy sources, and issues at the agency level to share with other stakeholders. Areas of uncertainty should be noted and clarified with partners.
- Refer back to the toolkit introduction (Chapter 3) for key definitions and concepts.

---

[3] The blank table for participants to complete can be downloaded from the project's website: www.iom.edu/crisisstandards.

Scope and Event Type: _____

Indicator Category	Contingency	Crisis	Return Toward Conventional
Surveillance data	Indicators: Triggers: Tactics:	Indicators: Crisis triggers: Tactics:	Indicators: Triggers: Tactics:
Communications and community infrastructure	Indicators: Triggers: Tactics:	Indicators: Crisis triggers: Tactics:	Indicators: Triggers: Tactics:
Staff	Indicators: Triggers: Tactics:	Indicators: Crisis triggers: Tactics:	Indicators: Triggers: Tactics:
Space/infrastructure	Indicators: Triggers: Tactics:	Indicators: Crisis triggers: Tactics:	Indicators: Triggers: Tactics:
Supplies	Indicators: Triggers: Tactics:	Indicators: Crisis triggers: Tactics:	Indicators: Triggers: Tactics:
Other categories	Indicators: Triggers: Tactics:	Indicators: Crisis triggers: Tactics:	Indicators: Triggers: Tactics:

REFERENCES

ASPR (Assistant Secretary for Preparedness and Response). 2012. *Hospital preparedness program (HPP) performance measure manual, guidance for using the new HPP performance measures.* Washington, DC: Department of Health and Human Services. http://www.phe.gov/Preparedness/planning/evaluation/Documents/hpp-coag.pdf (accessed June 5, 2013).

IOM (Institute of Medicine). 2012. *Crisis standards of care: A systems framework for catastrophic disaster response.* Washington, DC: The National Academies Press. http://www.nap.edu/openbook.php?record_id=13351 (accessed April 3, 2013).

A: Glossary[1]

Alternate care facility A temporary site, not located on hospital property, established to provide patient care. It may provide either ambulatory or nonambulatory care. It may serve to "decompress" hospitals that are maximally filled, or to bolster community-based triage capabilities. Has also been referred to as an "alternate care site."

Certain data Data that require minimal verification and analysis to initiate a trigger.

Clinical care committee Composed of clinical and administrative leaders at a health care institution, this committee is responsible for prioritizing the allocation of critical life-sustaining interventions. The clinical care committee may also be formed at the health care coalition level (e.g., hospital, primary care, emergency medical services agency, public health, emergency management, and others), playing the role of the disaster medical advisory committee at the regional level (see **disaster medical advisory committee**). May appoint a triage team (see **triage team**) to evaluate case-by-case decisions.

Contingency surge The spaces, staff, and supplies used are not consistent with daily practices, but provide care that is *functionally equivalent* to usual patient care practices. These spaces or practices may be used temporarily during a major mass casualty incident or on a more sustained basis during a disaster (when the demands of the incident exceed community resources).

Conventional capacity The spaces, staff, and supplies used are consistent with daily practices within the institution. These spaces and practices are used during a major mass casualty incident that triggers activation of the facility emergency operations plan.

Crisis standards of care The level of care possible during a crisis or disaster due to limitations in supplies, staff, environment, or other factors. These standards will usually incorporate the following principles: (1) prioritize population health rather than individual outcomes; (2) respect ethical principles of beneficence,

---

[1] The definitions provided in this glossary are from the 2012 report (IOM, 2012) with the inclusion of several new terms that are specifically addressed in this report.

stewardship, equity, and trust; (3) modify regulatory requirements to provide liability protection for health care providers making resource allocation decisions; and/or (4) designate a crisis triage officer and include provisions for palliative care in triage models for scarce resource allocation (e.g., ventilators). Crisis standards of care will usually follow a formal declaration or recognition by state government during a pervasive (pandemic influenza) or catastrophic (earthquake, hurricane) disaster which recognizes that contingency surge response strategies (resource-sparing strategies) have been exhausted, and crisis medical care must be provided for a sustained period of time. Formal recognition of these austere operating conditions enables specific legal/regulatory powers and protections for health care provider allocation of scarce medical resources and for alternate care facility operations. Under these conditions, the goal is still to supply the best care possible to each patient.

Crisis surge Adaptive spaces, staff, and supplies are not consistent with usual standards of care, but provide sufficiency of care in the setting of a catastrophic disaster (i.e., provide the best possible care to patients given the circumstances and resources available). Crisis capacity activation constitutes a *significant* adjustment to standards of care.

Disaster medical advisory committee At the state or regional level, evaluates evidence-based, peer-reviewed critical care and other decision tools and recommends decision-making algorithms to be used when life-sustaining resources become scarce. May also be involved in providing broader recommendations regarding disaster planning and response efforts. When formed at the regional level, this group may take on the same functions as that of the clinical care committee. Those functions are focused in two distinct areas—medical advisory input and resource allocation decision approval.

Emergency Management Assistance Compact (EMAC) The first national disaster-relief compact, the EMAC has been adopted by all 50 states and the District of Columbia. It uses a responsive system that connects states with each other and federal government agencies during governor-declared emergencies, allowing them to request and send personnel, equipment, and other resources to the site of disasters.

Emergency medical services (EMS) The full spectrum of emergency care, from recognition of the emergency, telephone access of the system, and provision of prehospital care, through definitive care in the hospital. It often also includes medical response to disasters, planning for and provision of medical coverage at mass gatherings, and interfacility transfers of patients. However, for the purposes of this document, the definition of EMS is limited to the more traditional, colloquial meaning: prehospital health care for patients with real or perceived emergencies from the time point of emergency telephone access until arrival and transfer of care to the hospital.

Emergency response system A formal or informal organization covering a specified geographic area minimally composed of health care institutions, public health agencies, emergency management agencies, and emergency medical services providers to facilitate regional preparedness planning and response.

Health care coalition A group of individual health care assets (e.g., hospitals, clinics, long-term care facilities, etc.) in a specified geographic location that have partnered to respond to emergencies in a coordinated manner. The coalition has both a preparedness element and a response organization that possess appropriate structures, processes, and procedures. During response, the goals of the coalition are to facilitate situational awareness, resource support, and coordination of incident management among the participating organizations.

Health care institution Any facility providing patient care. This includes acute care hospitals, community health centers, long-term care institutions, private practices, and skilled nursing facilities.

Health care practitioners Include "health care professionals" and other non-licensed individuals who are involved in the delivery of health care services.

Health care professionals Individuals who are licensed to provide health care services under state law.

Indicator A measurement, event, or other data that is a predictor of change in demand for health care service delivery or availability of resources. This may warrant further monitoring, analysis, information sharing, and/or select implementation of emergency response system actions.

- **Actionable indicator:** An indicator that *can* be impacted through actions taken within an organization or component of the emergency response system (e.g., a hospital detecting high patient census).
- **Predictive indicator:** An indicator that *cannot* be impacted through actions taken within an organization or component of the emergency response system (e.g., a hospital receiving notification that a pandemic virus has been detected).

Legal standard of care The minimum amount of care and skill that a health care practitioner must exercise in particular circumstances based on what a reasonable and prudent health care practitioner would do in similar circumstances; during non-emergencies and disasters, they are based on the specific situation.

Medical standard of care The type and level of medical care required by professional norms, professional requirements, and institutional objectives; these standards vary as circumstances change, including during emergencies or crisis events.

Memorandums of Understanding (MOUs) Voluntary agreements among agencies and/or jurisdictions for the purpose of providing mutual aid at the time of a disaster.

Mutual aid agreements (MAAs) Written instruments among agencies and/or jurisdictions in which they agree to assist one another on request by furnishing personnel and equipment. An "agreement" is generally more legally binding than an "understanding."

Non-scripted tactic A tactic that varies according to the situation; it is based on analysis, multiple or uncertain indicators, recommendations, and, in certain circumstances, previous experience.

Palliative care Care provided by an interdisciplinary team to prevent and relieve suffering and to support the best possible quality of life for patients and their families, regardless of the stage of the disease or the need for other therapies. Palliative care affirms life by supporting the patient and family's goals for the future, including their hopes for cure or life prolongation, as well as their hopes for peace and dignity throughout the course of illness, the dying process, and death.

Protocol A written procedural approach to a specific problem or condition.

Public health system A complex network of individuals, organizations, and relevant critical infrastructures that have the potential to act individually and together to create conditions of health, including communities, health care delivery systems (e.g., home care, ambulatory care, private practice, hospitals, skilled nursing facilities, and others), employers and business, the media, homeland security and public safety, academia, and the governmental public health infrastructure.

Region An organizational area defined for the purpose of efficiently coordinating, administering, and facilitating disaster preparedness, response, and recovery activities. The area is typically determined by geographic, jurisdictional, demographic, political, and/or functional service area boundaries. For example, it may be based on areas that are already established for activities conducted by public-sector partners (e.g., federal, state, local, or tribal governments), such as existing regions defined by public health, emergency management, EMS, or law enforcement agencies, or for activities conducted by private-sector partners, such as existing regions defined for delivering hospital and trauma care. The area may be within a state's boundaries (i.e., an intrastate region), including spanning substate jurisdictional lines (e.g., county and city lines); may cross state boundaries (i.e., an interstate region); or may be a hybrid (e.g., adjacent counties in bordering states). These factors also may be used to help define the boundaries of health care coalitions.

Regional Disaster Medical Advisory Committee (RDMAC) A designated group of subject matter experts who can homogenize state and local crisis care clinical guidance when the affected region encompasses areas across state lines. The RDMAC is necessary because state guidance alone may not address the specific needs of an area. Although regional guidance can provide greater clarity on applying state guidance in local situations, it must not be inconsistent with it. The RDMAC can also serve as the coordinator of information and process improvement where appropriate.

Resource sparing The process of maximizing the utility of supplies and material through conservation, substitution, reuse, adaptation, and reallocation.

Scope of practice The extent of a professional's ability to provide health services pursuant to their competence and license, certification, privileges, or other lawful authority to practice.

Scripted tactic A tactic that is predetermined (i.e., can be listed on a checklist) and is quickly implemented by frontline personnel with minimal analysis.

SOFA score The Sequential Organ Failure Assessment (SOFA) is a scoring system to determine the extent of a person's organ function or rate of failure. The score is based on six different body systems: respiratory, cardiovascular, hepatic, hematopoietic, renal, and neurologic.

State Disaster Medical Advisory Committee (SDMAC) The dedicated body within a state that is responsible, in planning for or during an emergency, for providing clinical and other crisis standards of care (CSC) guidance when prolonged or widespread crisis care is necessary to maintain a consistent basis for life-sustaining resource allocation decisions. During a response, the SDMAC should draw on the expertise of its membership and that of other preidentified subject matter experts to address ongoing issues as crisis care is implemented. The SDMAC's guidance should accompany other state declarations or invocations of emergency powers to empower and protect providers during their provision of crisis care.

Threshold "A level, point, or value above which something is true or will take place and below which it is not or will not" (Merriam-Webster Dictionary, 2013). A trigger point may be designed to occur at a threshold recognized by the community or agency to require a specific response. Trigger points and thresholds may be the same in many circumstances, but each threshold does not necessarily have an associated trigger.

Triage The process of sorting patients and allocating aid on the basis of need for or likely benefit from medical treatment. Types of triage include

- **Primary triage:** The first triage of patients into the medical system (it may occur out of hospital), at which point patients are assigned an acuity level based on the severity of their illness/disease.
- **Secondary triage:** Reevaluation of the patient's condition after initial medical care. This may occur at the hospital following EMS interventions or after initial interventions in the emergency department. This often involves the decision to admit the patient to the hospital.
- **Tertiary triage:** Further reevaluation of the patients' response to treatment after further interventions; this is ongoing during their hospital stay. This is the least practiced and least well-defined type of triage.

Triage team Appointed by the clinical care committee, uses decision tools appropriate to the event and resource being triaged, making tertiary triage using scarce resource allocation decisions. This is similar in concept to triage teams established to evaluate incoming patients to the emergency department requiring primary or secondary triage, usually in a sudden-onset, no-notice disaster event (e.g., explosive detonation).

Trigger Evidence that austere conditions prevail so that crisis standards of care practices will be required. This may occur at an institutional, and often regional, level of response. It suggests the need for the immediate implementation of response pathways that are required to manage a crisis surge response emanating from the disaster situation.

- **Crisis care trigger:** The point at which the scarcity of resources requires a transition from contingency care to crisis care, implemented within and across the emergency response system. This marks the transition point at which resource allocation strategies focus on the community rather than the individual.
- **Non-scripted:** A decision point that requires analysis and leads to implementation of non-scripted tactics.
- **Scripted trigger:** A predefined decision point that can be initiated immediately upon recognizing a qualifying indicator. Scripted triggers lead to scripted tactics.

Uncertain data Data that require interpretation to determine appropriate triggers and tactics.

REFERENCES

IOM (Institute of Medicine). 2012. *Crisis standards of care: A systems framework for catastrophic disaster response.* Washington, DC: The National Academies Press. http://www.nap.edu/catalog.php?record_id=13351.

Merriam-Webster Dictionary. 2013. *Definition of "threshold."* Springfield, MA: Encyclopaedia Britannica. http://www.merriam-webster.com/dictionary/threshold (accessed April 3, 2013).

B: Open Session Agenda

January 15, 2013

The National Academies
Keck Center, Room 110
500 Fifth Street, NW, Washington, DC 20001

OPEN SESSION 1: SPONSOR BRIEFING—BACKGROUND AND OVERVIEW

Session Objective: To obtain a better understanding of the background to the study and the charge to the committee.

11:00 a.m.   Welcome and Introductions

              DAN HANFLING, *Committee Co-Chair*
              Special Advisor, Emergency Preparedness and Response
              Inova Health System

              JOHN HICK, *Committee Co-Chair*
              Associate Medical Director for Emergency Medical Services and Medical Director of
                  Emergency Preparedness
              Hennepin County Medical Center

11:05 a.m.   Background and Charge to the Committee

              NICOLE LURIE
              Assistant Secretary for Preparedness and Response
               U.S. Department of Health and Human Services

11:30 a.m.   Working Lunch and Panel Discussion with Sponsors

GAMUNU WIJETUNGE
Office of Emergency Medical Services
National Highway Traffic Safety Administration
U.S. Department of Transportation

SHAYNE BRANNMAN
Senior Management Analyst
Office of the Assistant Secretary for Preparedness and Response
U.S. Department of Health and Human Services

12:30 p.m.   BREAK

OPEN SESSION 2: INDICATORS AND TRIGGERS ALONG THE CONVENTIONAL, CONTINGENCY, CRISIS CONTINUUM OF SURGE RESPONSE AND STANDARDS OF CARE

Session Objectives: To explore indicators and triggers for transitions along the continuum of care, from *conventional* to *contingency* to *crisis* surge capacity and standards of care, and back to *conventional* standards of care. Specifically,

- Identify potential indicators and triggers for different components of the emergency response system.
- Identify existing metrics for these indicators and triggers.
- Examine challenges that stakeholders would face in using these indicators and triggers to determine whether the health system should implement actions to avoid *contingency* or *crisis* surge capacity and standards of care plans and, later on, to determine when the health system should move back to *conventional* standards of care.
- Discuss the process through which stakeholders could work together to determine indicators and triggers for a specific jurisdiction. Identify successful multistakeholder processes that could serve as models for developing templates for multistakeholder discussions about indicators and triggers.

1:00 p.m.   Welcome and Introductions

DAN HANFLING, *Committee Co-Chair*
Special Advisor, Emergency Preparedness and Response
Inova Health System

JOHN HICK, *Committee Co-Chair*
Associate Medical Director for Emergency Medical Services and Medical Director of
    Emergency Preparedness
Hennepin County Medical Center

1:15 p.m.   Indicators and Triggers for Components of the Emergency Response System, Panel #1
    (Agencies and Coalitions)

DAN HANFLING, *Committee Co-Chair and Panel Moderator*

SUZET MCKINNEY
Deputy Commissioner
Bureau of Public Health Preparedness and Emergency Response
Chicago Department of Public Health

CYNTHIA DOLD
Healthcare Coalition Program Manager
Northwest Healthcare Response Network

JACK BROWN
Director
Arlington County Office of Emergency Management, Virginia

EDWARD TANZMAN
Codirector, Center for Integrated Emergency Preparedness
Decision and Information Sciences Division
Argonne National Laboratory

2:15 p.m.   Discussion with Committee Members, Speakers, and Attendees

3:00 p.m.   BREAK

3:15 p.m.   Indicators and Triggers for Components of the Emergency Response System, Panel #2
    (Health Care Entities and Specific Disciplines)

JOHN HICK, *Committee Co-Chair and Panel Moderator*

PEGGY CONNORTON
Director, Quality and LTC Trend Tracker
American Health Care Association

Barbara Citarella
President and CEO
RBC Limited Healthcare and Management Consultants

Gerard Jacobs
Professor of Psychology
Director, Disaster Mental Health Institute
University of South Dakota

Randy Kearns
State Burn Disaster Program Coordinator/Program Director/Researcher
North Carolina Jaycee Burn Center
University of North Carolina School of Medicine

4:15 p.m.   Discussion with Committee Members, Speakers, and Attendees

5:30 p.m.   ADJOURN

C: Committee Biosketches

Dan Hanfling, M.D. (*Co-Chair*), is special advisor to the Inova Health System in Falls Church, Virginia, on matters related to emergency preparedness and disaster response. He is a board-certified emergency physician practicing at Inova Fairfax Hospital, Northern Virginia's Level I trauma center. He serves as an operational medical director for air medical services and has responsibilities as a medical team manager for Virginia Task Force One, a Federal Emergency Management Agency (FEMA) and U.S. Agency for International Development sanctioned international urban search and rescue team. He has been involved in the response to the Izmit, Turkey, earthquake in 1999; the Pentagon in September 2001; and Hurricanes Rita and Katrina in 2005, and Gustav and Ike in 2008. He also participated in the response to the devastating earthquake in January 2010 near Port-au-Prince, Haiti. Dr. Hanfling was integrally involved in the management of the response to the anthrax bioterror mailings in the fall of 2001, when two cases of inhalational anthrax were successfully diagnosed and managed at Inova Fairfax Hospital. Dr. Hanfling is a founding member of the Northern Virginia Hospital Alliance. He has testified before Congress on the issues of disaster preparedness, and lectures nationally and internationally on prehospital-, hospital-, and disaster-related subjects. He served as vice chair of the Institute of Medicine (IOM) Committee on Establishing Standards of Care in Disaster Events. Dr. Hanfling received an A.B. in political science from Duke University, and was awarded his medical degree from Brown University. He completed an internship in internal medicine at the Miriam Hospital in Providence, Rhode Island, and an emergency medicine residency at George Washington/Georgetown University Hospitals. He is a clinical professor of emergency medicine at George Washington University, contributing scholar at the UPMC Center for BioSecurity, and adjunct distinguished senior fellow at the George Mason University School of Public Policy.

John L. Hick, M.D. (*Co-Chair*), is a faculty emergency physician at Hennepin County Medical Center (HCMC) and an associate professor of emergency medicine at the University of Minnesota. He serves as the associate medical director for Hennepin County Emergency Medical Services and as medical director for emergency preparedness at HCMC. He also serves the Minnesota Department of Health as the medical director for the Office of Emergency Preparedness. He is the founder and past chair of the Minneapolis/St. Paul Metropolitan Hospital Compact, a 30-hospital mutual aid and planning group active since 2002. He is involved at many levels of planning for surge capacity and crisis standards of care (CSC) and traveled to Greece to assist its health care system preparations for the 2004 Summer Olympics as part of a 15-member Centers for Disease Control and Prevention/Department of Health and Human Services (CDC/HHS) team. He has served as a member on IOM committees addressing crisis standards of care and is a national speaker on hospital preparedness issues. He has published numerous papers dealing with surge capacity, hospital preparedness for contaminated casualties, personal protective equipment, crisis care, and response to improvised nuclear device detonations.

Sarita Chung, M.D., is the director of disaster preparedness in the Division of Emergency Medicine at Boston Children's Hospital. Currently, she also serves on the Disaster Preparedness Advisory Council for the American Academy of Pediatrics and the National Advisory Council for FEMA. Trained in pediatrics and pediatric emergency medicine, Dr. Chung is actively involved in all aspects of pediatric emergency preparedness, including research, teaching, and clinical care. In terms of her research, Dr. Chung published one of the first post-9/11 articles, examining the efficacy of Web-based training in bioterrorism (at a time when such websites were proliferating, without evidence of their value) and showing that a Web-based educational tool does not enhance the knowledge of emergency physicians. She has gone on to publish important concept and research papers on issues of pediatric disaster preparedness such as the role of hospital preparation for disasters involving children, school preparedness, and reunification of children separated from their parents after a disaster. In terms of teaching, Dr. Chung is a nationally recognized lecturer on pediatric aspects of disaster preparedness, having presented at federally sponsored workshops and national pediatric meetings. She has also participated in national consensus conferences to discuss disaster preparedness for children. Dr. Chung is an assistant professor of pediatrics at Harvard School of Medicine.

Carol Cunningham, M.D., was appointed state medical director for the Ohio Department of Public Safety, Division of EMS, in July 2004 and is a board certified emergency physician at Akron General Medical Center and an assistant professor of emergency medicine at Northeast Ohio Medical University. She is the emergency medical services (EMS) medical director representative on the National EMS Advisory Council (NEMSAC) and the immediate past chairperson of the National Association of State EMS Officials (NASEMSO) Medical Directors Council. She also serves on Ohio's State Medical Coordination Committee. Dr. Cunningham received her M.D. and completed an emergency medicine residency at the University of Cincinnati. She has 7 years of experience as a flight physician and 11 years as a tactical EMS medical director, and is a fellow in the American College of Emergency Physicians and the American Academy of Emergency Medicine. Dr. Cunningham completed the National Preparedness Leadership Initiative at the Harvard Kennedy School of Executive Education and the Homeland Security Executive Leadership Program at The Naval Postgraduate School & The U.S. Department of Homeland Security Center for Homeland Defense and Security. She is the 2012 recipient of the American Academy of Emergency Medicine's James Keaney Leadership Award. Dr. Cunningham was appointed to the EMS Examination Task Force by the American Board of Emergency Medicine as an item writer for the EMS subspecialty examination in addition to her continued duties as an oral board examiner. She is a member of the editorial board of the *Journal of EMS*, a contributing editor for the *EMS Insider*, and an ad hoc member of the HHS Agency for Healthcare Research and Quality's Health Care Technology and Decision Science panel. Dr. Cunningham is the co–principal investigator for the Model EMS Clinical Guidelines project, and the NASEMSO physician representative working with the National Highway Traffic Safety Administration (NHTSA) on the

National EMS Education Standards Implementation Team. She also served as a member of the Education and Workforce Committee of the NEMSAC. She also serves on the EMS Program Steering Committee of the National Fire Academy Board of Visitors, the Department of Homeland Security (DHS) Science & Technology Directorate's First Responder Resource Group, and the EMS Support Team of the DHS/FEMA National Integration Center Strategic Resource Group.

Brian Flynn, Ed.D., is a consultant, writer, trainer, and speaker specializing in preparation for, response to, and recovery from the psychosocial aspects of large-scale emergencies and disasters. He has served numerous national and international organizations, states, and academic institutions. In addition, he currently serves as associate director of the Center for the Study of Traumatic Stress, and adjunct professor of psychiatry, Department of Psychiatry, Uniformed Services University of the Health Sciences, in Bethesda, Maryland. In 2002, he left federal service as a rear admiral/assistant surgeon general in the Public Health Service. He has directly operated, and supervised the operation of, the federal government's domestic disaster mental health program (including terrorism) and programs in suicide and youth violence prevention, child trauma, refugee mental health, women's and minority mental health concerns, and rural mental health. He has served as an adviser to many federal departments and agencies, states, and national professional organizations. He is recognized internationally for his expertise in large-scale trauma and has served as an adviser to practitioners, academicians, and government officials in many nations. He received his B.A. from North Carolina Wesleyan College, his M.A. in clinical psychology from East Carolina University, and his Ed.D. in mental health administration from the University of Massachusetts at Amherst.

W. Nim Kidd, CEM, was appointed to the position of assistant director for the Texas Department of Public Safety in 2010. He serves as the chief of the Texas Division of Emergency Management, responsible for the state's emergency preparedness, response, recovery, and mitigation activities. From 2004 to 2010, Chief Kidd served as the emergency manager and homeland security coordinator for the City of San Antonio. He managed the city's preparedness, response, and recovery efforts for all local disasters, including more than a dozen state, major, and presidential disaster declarations. He has been a member of the Texas Task Force 1 Urban Search and Rescue Team since 1997 and has responded to several state and national disasters, including the World Trade Center attack in September 2001.

Ann R. Knebel, Ph.D., R.N., FAAN, is the deputy director of the National Institute of Nursing Research. Dr. Knebel has been instrumental in advancing various preparedness planning and surge capacity initiatives. Highlights include developing publications that have had a national impact on preparedness such as a handbook on medical surge capacity and capability, and planning guidance on allocation of scarce resources. Dr. Knebel serves on expert panels that influence international approaches to preparedness, such as a World Health Organization–sponsored virtual advisory group on mass gathering preparedness. Dr. Knebel completed a doctorate of philosophy at the University of California, San Francisco. Her prior experiences include serving in both the intramural and the extramural programs at the National Institutes of Health, with a primary focus on advancing policy initiatives and developing research programs for symptom management, quality of life, and end-of-life issues. She is a fellow of the American Academy of Nursing.

Linda Scott, R.N., M.A., is the manager of the Healthcare Preparedness Program in the Office of Public Health Preparedness at the Michigan Department of Community Health. She is responsible for coordinating the HHS Assistant Secretary for Preparedness and Response Hospital Preparedness Program working in collaboration with CDC Public Health Emergency Preparedness activities. Ms. Scott holds a B.S. in nursing and an M.A. in homeland security studies from the Naval Postgraduate School.

Anthony H. Speier, Ph.D., is a developmental psychologist. He was trained at the University of Texas in Austin and Louisiana State University. Dr. Speier is assistant secretary for the Office of Behavioral Health in the state of Louisiana's Department of Health and Hospitals. Before this, he served as the director of Disaster Mental Health Operations for the Louisiana Office of Mental Health, in which capacity he was the principal contact for all federally funded crisis counseling programs addressing the emotional impact of Hurricane Katrina on Louisiana residents. Dr. Speier formerly served as the director of the Division of Program Development and Implementation for the Louisiana Office of Mental Health. He also led the Office of Mental Health Substance Abuse and Mental Health Services Administration Co-Occurring State Incentive Grant project and has been the principal investigator on a number of Center for Mental Health Services (CMHS) systems change grants focusing on issues specific to adults with severe and persistent mental illness. In his capacity as the state director for disaster mental health coordination and response activities, Dr. Speier has been the project director for nine federal crisis counseling grants following presidentially declared disasters in Louisiana. He has served as chair of the Adult Services Division of the National Association of State Mental Health Program Directors. He is a practicing psychologist in Louisiana and holds a clinical appointment at the Louisiana State University Health Sciences Center Department of Psychiatry. Dr. Speier has authored a number of publications and training manuals for the CMHS.

Jolene R. Whitney, **M.P.A.,** is currently deputy director for the Utah Bureau of EMS and Preparedness, and has served as the state trauma system program manager for more than 20 years. She supervises 22 staff performing various functions related to trauma system development (including stroke and ST-elevation myocardial infarction [STEMI]), chemical stockpile emergency preparedness, surge capacity and MCI planning, emergency department, trauma and prehospital databases, EMS licensing and operations, certification and testing processes, critical incident stress management, National Disaster Medical System, EMS medical disaster resources, and the EMS for Children program. She has worked with the Bureau of Emergency Medical Services and Preparedness, Utah Department of Health, for more than 32 years. Ms. Whitney earned her M.P.A. from Brigham Young University and a B.S. in health sciences, with an emphasis in community health education, from the University of Utah. She was certified as an Emergency Medical Technician (EMT) basic in 1979 and obtained certification as an EMT instructor and EMT III (intermediate) in 1983. She has attended numerous conferences, courses, and workshops on EMS, trauma, and disaster planning and response (ICS 100, 200, 300, 700, and 800). Ms. Whitney is a coauthor of six publications pertaining to domestic violence, preventable trauma mortality, Western states rural care challenges, and state and hospital surge capacity planning. Ms. Whitney recently served as an IOM Crisis Standards of Care Committee member in the development of the System Framework for Catastrophic Disaster Response. She also served on the Workshop Planning Committee and as panel chair for the IOM Preparedness and Response to a Rural Mass Casualty Incident Workshop. Ms. Whitney has participated on several national committees and teams, which include state EMS system assessments for NHTSA (Delaware, Michigan, Missouri, Ohio, and Oklahoma), American College of Surgeons trauma system assessments (Alaska, Colorado, Louisiana, Minnesota, and Texas), and Health Resources and Services Administration (HRSA) rural trauma grant reviews. She contributed to the development of the HRSA model trauma system plan, the NASEMSO trauma system planning guide, the National Trauma Data Standards, and the NHTSA curriculum for an EMT refresher course. She is the previous past chair for the National Council of State Trauma System Managers/NASEMSO and served as vice chair for the previous 3 years. She is a member of the American Trauma Society and the Utah Emergency Managers Association. Previously she was a member of the National Association of State EMS Training Coordinators and Utah Public Health Association. Ms. Whitney spent 250 hours in the Olympic Command Center, serving as a hospital liaison for the 2002 Winter Olympics in Salt Lake City. Ms. Whitney is currently assisting with the development of Utah-1 Disaster Medical Assistance Team and has recently been hired as a federal intermittent employee for the team, and serves as the acting planning section chief.